# What Is Fat For?

## Re-Thinking Obesity Science

**Ignatius Brady MD, MPH**

*—Iowa City—*

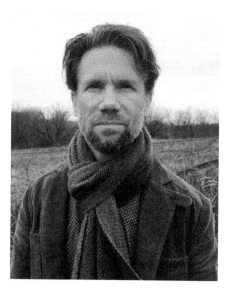

Ignatius Brady is a physician who lives and practices in Iowa. He has worked in corporate health, wellness, quality improvement, weight management, and most recently, with the Veteran's Hospital in Iowa City. He is a featured writer on Science 2.0, where he covers topics related to metabolism, nutrition, and public health. He is available for lectures and readings. For information regarding his availability, please contact: Outreach@whatisfatfor.com

Disclaimer: While the author is a medical doctor and the topics covered in this text touch upon new approaches for medical conditions, there is no expressed or implied professional advice herein. Readers are advised that Chapter 7 contains important reservations regarding the application of the book's insights. *Do not stop medications without medical advice.* Discuss any and all dietary changes with your dietitian and physician.

ISBN: 978-0-692-59006-5  1. Obesity. 2. Nutrition. 3. Physiology. 4. Energy metabolism. 5. Weight loss.

Available from Amazon.com, Createspace.com, and other retail outlets.

# Contents

# Preface

*"Most obese persons will not stay in treatment. Of those who stay in treatment, most will not lose weight, and of those who do lose weight, most will regain it."*

—*Mickey Stunkard, MD 1958*

Dr. Stunkard passed on this accumulated wisdom from advising and studying obese patients for over a decade. It did not deter him from working on a disease that he found fascinating, and he continued to study and publish on the subject for 50 more years after the above quotation. About a decade ago, I was lucky enough to hear him speak about why he was inspired to work on this disease which refused to be cured. I left his talk enthused by the many aspects of the obese condition that he found open to fresh insights and in need of interested clinicians. A decade later, my own experience working with patients has convinced me that what was true in 1958 is true today: Medical doctors can do very little to help patients lose weight.

This is not an occasional observation. The journals repeatedly publish reviews and meta-analyses of diet studies. Even under the optimum conditions of a controlled trial (motivated individuals, strict selection criteria, multidisciplinary teams of observers and helpers, frequent follow up, adequate funding) average weight losses generally run 2 to 20 pounds (~1 to 9 kg) at the one year point. The vast majority of the results are closer to the 2 than the 20, and patients are almost universally on the upswing at the time of last follow up, suggesting that they tend to gain back all the weight lost. Studies of commercial programs, which operate without the depth of wisdom available to physician-led programs, do even worse. Weight Watchers is the only widely available commercial program to have published results in a peer-reviewed journal, and they were found to produce exactly zero pounds of weight loss on average at one year. We might speculate that the other programs, which have not dared to publish, are doing worse still, perhaps with participants on average *gaining,* rather than losing weight.

More important than the average results of the average study is the almost incredible fact that no study published to date is an outlier. Outside of the literature on bariatric surgery, there simply are no studies showing participants losing consistently 30 pounds (~13 kg) or more at one year. This is despite all the advantages mentioned above regarding studies. That they produce what you might call negligible weight loss after selecting the participants so carefully makes one wonder how patients might be doing under usual care. Very few weight loss studies enroll patients with diabetes, let alone depression, kidney failure, heart disease, serious orthopedic restrictions, or the just plain weird folks who are a part of the real world. Despite this, we physicians generally walk around with the notion that we are doing a lot of good in our weight loss practice . . . never running a trial of our own. We assume, strangely, that we somehow must be doing better than the average, despite our skeleton staff, complex patient mix and lack of funding. Generally, we ascribe our presumed (never measured) superior results to our presumed (never measured) superior knowledge of how obesity works.

George A. Bray, a prominent obesity scientist and clinician, wrote a history of obesity research and diet treatments dating back to ancient times called *The Battle of the Bulge*. He points out that there seem to be only three weight loss ideas: low-fat, low-carbohydrate, and low-calorie. Scientists, doctors and dietitians are in perpetual debate as to which of the three is correct. The low-calorie/mathematical advocates have the soundest scientific explanation for their view, since math and physics trump the other sciences (you never hear a biologist say to a physicist, "Well, that just doesn't fit with what we know about biology," but you do hear the reverse). Generally, low-calorie diet advocates presume that the balance of macronutrients we are eating now is adequate and that we can keep the same diet composition while simply eating less of everything. Most doctors sum this up in the not-so-illuminating directive: Eat less and exercise more. The other two diet concepts are based on the principal that there must be a primary cause of obesity, other than, or in addition to, calories. If too much fat in the diet causes us to grow fat cells, then we must reduce it. If too much carbohydrate is the culprit, then we must cut carbs instead. These two competing hypotheses rest on very different proposals for the pathway leading to fat storage. What they have in common is the belief that the calories themselves are not the correct target for intervention. Caloric intake is considered to be elevated as an accidental byproduct of bad choices and it will take care of itself after the nutritional imbalance is corrected.

The evolutionary biologist E.O. Wilson proposes, in his 1978 book *On Human Nature,* that scientific knowledge expands most effectively when the researchers in various fields become more aware of the discipline "above" and "below" their own. Cell biologists understanding chemistry "below" and physiology of the entire organism "above" their own scientific discipline would be an example. I believe that much of the debate regarding obesity causation is unnecessary and is due to just such a lack of awareness among the best scientists. While the debate between the low-carb advocates and the low-fat advocates plays out at the level of physiology, the mathematicians are focused on the energy balance of the entire animal. Researchers looking at our food supply and the greater nutritional environment are focused one level higher than the organism, the population. Their insights are very difficult to imagine impacting the metabolism of a single cell. Very few scientists who look at the energy balance in molecular terms, that is, anything smaller than a cell, are involved in the obesity debates at all.

I work as a medical doctor, which to say, in a field that exists to *apply* the insights of those other disciplines as they relate to human health. Physicians are neither above nor below the other disciplines, but simply outside of them altogether. Once you are done with your training, you can practice medicine using very little science, if you so choose. Applying the best practices advocated by respected authorities will keep patients safe and to do this does not require detailed knowledge of underlying mechanisms. More to the point, possessing more scientific knowledge does not necessarily make you a better physician. In my own case, I can say that it matters little to a weight loss patient whether I believe his obesity is due to changes in the agouti-related peptide regulation in his brain or increased secretion of ghrelin from the stomach, if I can't give him a pill or a strategy that affects either. Certainly, the small signaling pathways within cells, or the nuanced balance of neuropeptides in the hypothalamus do not even register for the average clinician. For some reason, when it comes to weight issues, physicians are as prone to using anecdotes as everyone else and frequently give weight loss advice based on what they've read in a popular magazine, or what's worked for them personally. We would never do that in other fields of medicine, but perfectly good clinicians lose their objectivity when it comes to weight issues. Thus far, the science of obesity and what happens in a primary care or a weight loss practice remain disconnected. Without drugs or strategies to translate the lab science to our practices, we are left with trial and error medicine. With this in mind, I don't feel confident enough that my years as a weight loss doctor qualify me to call this book a *synthesis* of the important discoveries of obesity science. But it is at least a *collection* of many under-appreciated insights available to an inquisitive mind with access to the medical literature and some small acquaintance with the scientists who are making progress in our understanding. This is presented with the appropriate degree of skepticism that comes from working with real patients with serious problems related to their weight.

Which diet is best for weight loss may not actually be the most interesting question we can ask, or try to answer, with regard to obesity. Philip Scherer and Roger Unger have proposed an alternative understanding of what the fat cells do for the human body. Using the word "lipotoxicity" to describe the effect of circulating fatty acids in the blood and tissues, they argue that the fat tissue in our bodies cannot be considered as simply problematic, something to be rid of, since its main function is to absorb the excess energy that we eat before it can do damage to our organs. In their view, the activities performed by the adipose compartment are vital to good health. With that in mind, our concept of what it means to gain weight, or to be obese, may need to be altered.

Bariatric surgery, particularly gastric bypass, is the only intervention which produces consistent, profound weight loss results that can last for decades. There is simply no comparing outcomes between dieting and surgery when it comes to weight. But more important than this is what the surgery does for type 2 diabetes. Studies repeatedly show that long term improvement or remission of diabetes is commonplace, even to be expected, after gastric bypass. Whether one feels that surgery is a too drastic method or not, this forces us to reconsider what type 2 diabetes actually *is*. If it can be reversed effectively, consistently, fairly immediately by a surgical procedure, then it is a different disease than the one we generally describe. Elevated blood sugar can be presumed to be more a symptom of food-body interactions gone awry than a progressive disease requiring lifelong medication. Combined with Scherer's idea of lipotoxicity, we can argue that both type 2 diabetes and obesity can be understood better if we consider them adaptive responses to the environment rather than disease states. This takes our discussion to its highest level, that of ecology.

If there is a unifying or synthesizing concept in the book, it is discussed in Chapter 4, which deals with protein leverage. I suggest that Stephen Simpson and David Raubenheimer have actually "solved" the problem of obesity causation and that utilizing their framework could go a long way toward reversing the process. It is fortuitous that their proposals don't require disproving any of the three existing hypotheses for obesity causation. While they don't address the debate directly, their protein leverage hypothesis reinforces that calories matter, fats matter, carbohydrates matter, but not for the reasons the advocates propose. Through very simple math, they suggest that protein in the diet, rather than the other nutrients, regulates our body composition. This is not to say that they suggest a high-protein weight loss solution. There is a reason why their 2012 book, *The Nature of Nutrition*, is not called *The Protein Leverage Diet*, which certainly would have sold more copies. Dietary balance, which is the core concept of the protein leverage framework, is a key for behaviorally sustainable dietary changes. To cast this complex balance as a simple "protein is good" message would miss the bigger picture: Obesity arises as a reaction to our nutritional environment.

Reconsidering the problem of obesity in ecological terms, maintaining that our current body shape is the manifestation of an adaptation to our environment, might suggest that the chapters toward the end of the book will recommend we build more bicycle paths. As much as I like them for my commute to work, I do not believe that bicycle paths will save us, or that the built environment is an important contributor to obesity rates. I will present the ecologic argument entirely from the perspective of what has changed in our food over the last forty years. Staying with this premise, I hope to show that there is good reason to believe that the oft-maligned "food industry" may ultimately reverse the obesity trend and that the reversal may already have begun. While we wait for changes in the food supply to fully manifest, I will argue that our understanding of the risk of being obese is misinformed and that there is every reason to expect a long life, even if our body shape is not exactly what we would prefer.

This is not a diet book. I don't have a universal prescription that will help you become "rock hard in 30 days" or anything of that sort. In fact, much of the book is dedicated to understanding why universal prescriptions don't tend to help us. This is a book about obesity written from the perspective of a physician who has struggled to make sense of the experience of his patients in light of the available medical literature. While there are very few patient stories included in the pages that follow, this is not to discount the important personal character of obesity medicine, or how much I feel I've gained from the patients with whom I've been privileged to work. My preference for examining obesity in the aggregate, in populations and within generic concepts of "human bodies," comes from a search for the truth about weight regulation. Anecdotes about what worked for an individual patient might be interesting, but it's critical to look at the group, if we want to generalize our observations. Too much of our attention in the public discussion of weight issues is focused on remarkable results that occur only occasionally and not enough interest is trained on the fact that, for nearly all individuals, obesity is lifelong.

Weight problems emerge in a realm that is largely outside of individual choice. Like any animal, humans are driven to eat by biological cues. We must eat in the environment in which we find ourselves at any given time. We happen to be an animal with a lot of ideas and emotions about our eating, but I don't think those ideas and emotions are crucial for understanding why our weight is currently increasing. As we show that obesity is caused by biological mechanisms responding to ecological cues, rather than gluttony and sloth, we move the discussion away from behavior and toward population health. This frames the discussion of what can be done in a much more positive light than insisting on finding a means to change our basic human nature and appetites. By addressing the universal failure of diet solutions and turning our attention to our eating environment, we stop trying to do the impossible and focus on what must inevitably change if we are ever to reverse the current obesity trend.

# Chapter 1

## Regulation of Human Body Weight

Let us start with nothing. A naive human has come to stay in your home. Perhaps it's a Tarzan type of character, just arrived from the wild, or, if you like a modern twist, it's a government agent who has been hit over the head and can't even remember his name. In any case, this naive human will, within a few hours of arrival, make his way to your kitchen and begin poking around, because he's hungry.

So let's start by recognizing this: Hunger is universal. How we modern, complicated, guilty, preoccupied people talk about hunger may sometimes confuse the point ("I just eat mindlessly"), but let us start with the fact that hunger exists.

He's hungry, but, for what? Let's hypothesize that the food is extremely unrecognizable to him. He's a particularly primitive Tarzan or the blow to the head was quite heavy. He takes the olive oil out of the cupboard and begins to drink it down, straight from the bottle. Within a swallow or two, he's gagging and spitting out the recommended healthy oil. Next, he spies the sugar bowl, sniffs and finds it pleasing. He tilts the container to his face and tries a mouthful. His mouth dries; he can barely swallow, but manages. It's an appealing flavor, but it's not food. He couldn't repeat that swallow again without feeling the gag reflex return. He tries again with butter —gag. Saltshaker —gag. Maple syrup —gag. What's going on?

It is a commonly stated notion, that we are trained to seek salt, sugar and fat by some evolutionary process. We sometimes consider ourselves to be actually "addicted" to these three flavors. But as we've just demonstrated with our naive human, we need these flavors in a certain balance, in particular amounts, with particular textures and densities. Our preference, actually more than preference, our primitive survival-oriented, instinctive reaction to food is to want a very highly designated type of nutrition. We may think that our eating behavior is driven by marketing and what our mothers have taught us, but there is a more fundamental regulator than those: our own body.

The body not only helps us distinguish "food" from "not food," but will also sort good food from bad, fresh from rotten, nutritious from toxic. As in the case of the oil, sugar, and salt, the body knows not only what we need, but also the right quantity and concentration. This protects us from too much of a good thing. One could build up from this simple example (we won't) to a discussion of all types of foods and the means by which the body attempts to get what it needs from Coke and Doritos. But to begin our present discussion, we need only to acknowledge that hunger exists and that what, and how much, we eat is regulated. The purpose of this regulation is to optimize function and ensure reproduction, but it seems also to be related to the overall size of the body. For the same reason we don't find ants the size of dogs, we don't see humans 2 cm or 4 meters tall. Regarding weight, we don't see adults who weigh 20 pounds, nor 2000 pounds. We can debate which parameters drive the regulation of human body size and appetite, but we cannot debate that the regulation exists to help our bodies remain within a certain range of optimum. It's impossible to think of any animal existing without mechanisms to produce a certain size and shape.

## Normal Weight Gain

In medical school one day, I heard something in a lecture that caught my interest. A professor mentioned that the natural progression of weight gain in adults happened to be almost exactly one pound (0.45 kg) per year. It was considered normal, he said, for adults to put on about 40 pounds from age 20 to 60. This had been a stable finding over the previous hundred years or so, the time frame for which we had weights for large enough groups of people to make such an observation. At that time, I happened to be 26 years old and weighed 126 pounds. The thought occurred to me that I'd be a good subject to test this hypothesis: Whatever age I was throughout my adult life, plus 100 more pounds, should tell me my weight. Being naturally "skinny," I didn't focus on my body weight much, stepping on a scale only when required at a doctor's visit. I went through various career stages, including insane hours in the hospital, eating cafeteria food and losing sleep.

Vacations, graduations, fathering children, moving houses six or seven times . . . I noticed at age 32, I weighed 132 pounds. I was a bit squishy at that time, so I

3

got back into the gym, began to lift weights, and drank protein shakes. At age 35, I weighed 135. Later, having a bit more free time available, I continued the weight lifting and resumed soccer and running. I had surgery on my knee and couldn't do aerobic exercise for many months. Some years I commuted by car, others by bike. I spent 12 years as a vegetarian, five years as a purposeful protein eater, a few more indulging in Sour Patch Kids and beer. With some of these changes, my weight would seem to rise or fall quickly over a few months, perhaps as much as 10 pounds, hiding the true steady trend. At age 45, as I write this, my weight sits squarely at 145 pounds.

I happened to develop an interest in obesity in the middle of my career and I never noticed a reference for that professor's contention of what is normal weight gain and never saw it repeated. However, in 2013, a group of researchers from Duke published "Young Adult Weight Trajectories Through Midlife by Body Mass Category." In this study, they used data from 10,000 individuals (aged 25-33) involved in a different longitudinal study, who happened to be weighed yearly, to get a sense of what is "normal" for adult weight gain. Remarkably, their data almost perfectly corroborated my professor's contention (and my own experience).

On average, these 10,000 adults gained 1.17 pounds (0.53 kg) per year. The researchers broke down the participants by body mass category and found that, whether one was skinny or heavy at the start of the study, more than 98% of the men and 92% of the women followed a trajectory that sloped upward. Let's put this another way: You could tell a 25 year old man with decent confidence that there is a 98% chance he is going to be gaining weight over the next 20 years. The Duke researchers referenced previous work by Dariush Mozaffarian in 2011, which showed an average adult weight increase of 0.84 pounds (0.38 kg) per year. If we take these two papers together, which used different populations and different methods, we come to the, rather convenient, rule that adult humans are "designed" to gain a pound per year.

This pound-per-year rule complicates the discussion of "set points" and "homeostasis." We spend much time trying to figure out what's wrong with the "homeostasis" of the human animal trying to remain at a stable weight, but forget that weight is almost never stable. It rises from the moment we are born until our very last decades. At the University of Colorado, researchers led by Dan Bessesen looked at these normal weight trajectories and tested what happens when you experimentally knock healthy humans off their slow steady weight gain paths.

They did the same with lab rats, after observing that gradual weight gain is the norm for rats who are allowed to eat as much as desired, just like humans. What they found was that when either humans or rats are deliberately overfed or underfed, the tendency, after the intervention ceases, is to return, not to the previous weight, but to the expected, slightly higher, weight predicted on the pound-per-year trajectory (and the grams per week equivalent for rats). This explains the near constant observation by patients that they dieted for a period of time, lost weight, then gained it all back "and a little more." In this case, the lead author suggests the use of the term "homeorrhesis" in lieu of homeostasis. The "rhesis" suffix denoting not *stability*, but a constant *trend* with a predictable direction. For

5

obesity, the question is not, "Why am I gaining weight?" but rather, "Why am I gaining *so much* weight?"

We are told that 1/3 of adults in the U.S. can be considered "overweight" and another third "obese." Those exact numbers and their true significance can be debated (and will be in Chapter 10), but we cannot argue with the fact that there is a significant portion of the population that would be considered, by nearly anyone, as having trouble regulating their body size.

If it is becoming more common than not that adults are dysregulated, the natural inclination would be to look for the cause of this dysregulation. Since the problem is so widespread, it seems likely that it is caused by a factor that is outside of our individual control. The possibility that the obesity epidemic has been caused by a massive, collective, sudden loss of will power in all industrialized nations, simultaneously, seems unlikely to me. In order to understand why obesity is rising, we need to look deeper into how our metabolism is regulated.

**Metabolism Is Variable**

A very perceptive group of researchers headed by Rudolph Liebel examined this issue in 1984. The paper appeared in the February issue of *Metabolism* and was titled "Diminished Energy Requirements in Reduced-Obese Patients."

What they wanted to know was this: Are heavy people who say they don't eat much totally full of crap? Well, they didn't quite phrase it that way, but they investigated the apparent phenomena of weight plateaus and regain patterns by asking: Do people actually need less food than expected after they've lost weight? Do their bodies somehow compensate and simply survive on less food? This is what many patients claim. But is it true?

It turns out it is, quite clearly, true. As the authors mention themselves, their methods were decidedly low-tech. This was a retrospective analysis of data gathered on the most successful participants of previous liquid diet trials at their institution. In the weight loss program, they checked volunteers into a hospital ward and prepared all of their meals with analyzed calorie counts, carefully measured ingredients and weighed all amounts eaten and left-over.

Letting the study subjects self-select food quantity and weighing them daily, Drs. Leibel and Hirsch calculated how many calories lean and obese subjects needed to maintain their baseline weight.

The first surprise: "The obese and control subjects required comparable caloric intakes."

Then, they analyzed what happened after the use of an aggressive meal replacement liquid diet of 600 calories/day which produced a very large weight loss in the treatment group. They then stabilized the participants at the new weight (50 kg less!) and calculated how much food was needed to keep them steady at the lower weight.

The second surprise: "Following weight loss, the reduced-obese subjects required only 1021 +/- 32 kcal/m$^2$ per day, a 28% decrease compared to their obese state and a 24% decrease relative to the control patients."

The third surprise: "The mean individual energy requirement of the reduced-obese subjects (2171 kcal/day) was less than that for the control subjects (2280 kcal/day) despite the fact that they still weighed 60% more than the controls." In the understated tone typical of good science, the authors concluded, "This finding has implications with regard to the pathophysiology and treatment of obesity in humans."

I'll say it has implications. Obese and lean people eat the same amount? Obese people need 28% fewer calories after weight loss? Obese people have to eat less than people who are much lighter than them, just to keep weight off? These findings have enormous implications for how we think about obesity and they don't seem to be common knowledge among clinicians. In fact, I hear most physician colleagues give the exact opposite opinion to their patients: that metabolisms *don't* vary. When did a doctor or a trainer or a dietitian ever tell a client that he might lose a great deal of weight, still be quite heavy and have to eat less than a skinny person, forever, to maintain that weight loss?

These conclusions regarding the needed caloric intake for those who have successfully lost weight are reinforced by data from the National Weight Control Registry, which is run by Rena Wing, from Brown University with James Hill, Holly Wyatt, and colleagues at the University of Colorado School of Medicine. They created the registry after realizing that so few people are successful with long term weight loss, it might be fruitful to just ask the exceptions, those that actually keep weight off long term, what they do that seems to be working.

In order to be included in the ongoing surveys and studies, participants must have lost at least 30 pounds and kept it off for a year. The average participant in the group has actually lost 60 pounds and kept it off for five years. With regard to calories, the women report eating just 1300 calories per day and the men, 1600. This corroborates the findings from Leibel and Hirsch: People who have lost weight need to eat much less than the naturally lean, if they are to keep the weight off.

In 1995, as a follow up to their 1984 study regarding reduced calorie requirements after weight loss, Leibel and Hirsch looked at a different group of lean and obese subjects. In this study, "Changes in Energy Expenditure Resulting from Altered Body Weight," they looked at how the body reacts to weight *gain,* in addition to weight *loss.* By systematically overfeeding or underfeeding the volunteers, they were able to show that all of the study subjects altered energy expenditure in such a manner as to bring the body back to its starting weight. When they overfed the subjects to cause a weight gain of 10%, the metabolism sped up in an attempt to burn off the excess. When they reduced the subjects by 10%, the metabolism slowed down to compensate. The increase that occurred after weight gain was more than expected for the increase in body mass. The decrease in metabolism was more than expected from the loss of body mass. With both interventions, the body was found to be *over-compensating* to fight its way back to normal. These same researchers went on to show, in 2008, "this disproportionate decline in [energy expenditure] persists after dynamic weight loss has ended . . . regardless of whether that reduced weight has been maintained for weeks or years."

Not every study that has looked for the phenomenon of slow metabolism after weight loss has agreed with the Leibel/Hirsch findings. Drs. Wyatt and Hill, whose registry suggests such very low maintenance calorie requirements when subjects self-report, went on to try to validate this more scientifically. They reported in an *American Journal of Clinical Nutrition* article in 1999, that the subjects they had actually brought in for metabolic testing were indistinguishable from a control group. So this suggests that the weight registry participants' reports of eating 1300-1600 calories per day may be a case of under-reporting.

However, when it comes to the proposition of whether it's possible that metabolism is slower after weight loss, we do not have to prove the phenomenon to be universal. Rather, we need only to show that it is *possible*. If it occurs in some (and this *does* seem to be the case from the studies mentioned above), we need to change our thinking. Previously, physicians had denied the possibility that individuals can vary with regard to core metabolic parameters. But since there seems to be ample evidence that the body slows down to conserve energy in response to weight loss, it's critical that the professionals counseling patients recognize this and the difficulties facing a person trying for long term changes in body shape and health. Patients have generally been misguided by their physicians. Because there is no specific lab test for metabolism (short of the very expensive, complicated procedures in the academic studies) physicians are generally unaware of the variability of these factors. Patients are usually told that there is no biological reason that they can't lose weight and maintain that loss. The underlying message, from the medical establishment, seems to be that obesity is the result of gluttony and sloth and that an individual's inability to get lighter is due to a lack of willpower.

The science simply doesn't back this up (in fact, the willpower nucleus in the brain has yet to be found). But patients have been so trained to blame themselves and told so often that their metabolism is normal (by physicians) that they can spend a lifetime trying to achieve something that may be, for all practical purposes, impossible: maintaining meaningful weight loss.

## Why True Weight Loss Is Rare

When you are a weight loss doctor, your friends and colleagues cannot help but comment on your work. Many conversations contain the question, "Isn't it all just . . . carbs, laziness, fast food, inactivity, genes, fructose —fill in speculation here." I began to avoid the subject of my job like it was a dirty little secret, but it came up fairly regularly nonetheless. Of the many completely wrong-headed things that non-obese people wonder, the one that I was asked most often was, "How does a person let themselves get that way?"

To really respond to that question would have required a discussion as long as this chapter, but my quick response was, "People don't *let* themselves get any particular way at all. You didn't *let* yourself get to be 6 feet tall or 200 pounds; your body decided that for you. A person with a serious weight problem has almost always spent a tremendous amount of effort struggling to get skinnier. If weight loss was a matter of deciding to change, we would not have obesity at all. A heavy person, walking around in our judgmental, body-conscious society, is living proof that we cannot decide our own weight."

What we know from trials that are published in medical journals is that we when we lose weight, the body will adapt. It does this through changes in our metabolic rate and also by changing hormones that are involved in energy balance. The idea that hormones control our body composition is not new. Defects in growth hormone, estrogen, and insulin have been recognized for nearly 100 years. But interest by researchers is increasing as the number of hormones identified as playing a role in weight regulation has grown considerably in the last two decades, with the current count at least 25.

With regard to searching for a signal that might alter weight regulation, the hormone most studied is leptin, a chemical that is made primarily in adipose tissue. Leptin is generally considered to be a "stop eating" signal to the brain. The amount of leptin in the circulation is proportional to the size of the adipose tissue, so, in the simplest of worlds, leptin could be a very good candidate for the main regulator of our size over long periods of time. As we grow larger, the quantity of leptin grows with us, telling the brain areas responsible for feeding: "Hey, we are big enough down here; it's okay to eat a little less."

The possibility that leptin was the key regulator of weight was first suggested by the fact that replacing the hormone in people who were born with a defective gene (they were remarkably large, even as toddlers) permanently relieved them of their obesity. Initial excitement about giving other obese patients leptin for weight loss died down quickly in the late 1990s, when it was found to be of no help to those with a normal leptin gene. Obese subjects without this rare genetic defect, in fact, make more leptin than their lean peers. Heavier people seem to become less responsive to the signal leptin sends over time, so this does not seem to be something we can override by giving more.

Acting in coordination and counterbalance to leptin's signal to eat less, are a host of hormonal signals. Among the most important is ghrelin, which is secreted from the stomach when it's empty. In addition to the nerves which respond to stretch signals in the stomach and intestines, the ghrelin secreting cells are actually responsive to the sugar, protein, and fat in the food that we eat.

Ghrelin tells the brain when the nutrients in the stomach are running low and sends a signal to the hypothalamus, encouraging an "eat more" response. There are other important hormonal signals, such as amylin from the pancreas, as well as CCK, GLP-1 and peptide YY from the intestine, which all sense nutrients flowing through the gut and report back to the brain on the feeding status of the body. When we "go on a diet," we are purposely underfeeding nutrients to this regulatory system. This does not go unnoticed. The signaling that ensures that humans survive through all manner of nutrient environments exists to adapt to these changes. It does so by altering the amounts of these gut and organ hormones to reverse deficiency when food becomes available.

In a study by Priya Sumathrin in 2011 entitled, "Long-Term Persistence of Hormonal Adaptations to Weight Loss," the researchers sought to quantify these hormonal changes by measuring blood hormone levels of 50 volunteers while they lost weight. The dietary intervention lasted 10 weeks and the method was to use a very low-calorie diet (~500 calories/day). The researchers successfully reduced the participants to 10% less than their original weight, 25-30 pounds (11-13 kg) on average. The hormones studied included leptin and ghrelin. They found that, as the study subjects became lighter, the hormones responded exactly as one might expect: The leptin (eat less) signal decreased and the ghrelin (eat more) signal increased, in an apparent effort to drive the body back to the baseline weight. Several of the hormones, including leptin, CCK and amylin, remained abnormal for *at least a year*, confirming that the hormones match the metabolic findings of Liebel and Hirsch. The authors concluded that these hormone changes support the view of a body weight set point and that the hormonal adaptations help to explain the generally abysmal rates of permanent weight loss produced by dieting.

If you want to get your doctor quickly worried about you, try mentioning that you've been gradually losing weight unintentionally. The reaction will be a long procession of general health questions, a very thorough exam, followed by a battery of tests looking for an undetected chronic illness such as cancer. People *do not* accidentally waste away. We never see it outside of illness. It makes sense that, when the normal upward weight trend is disrupted by our deliberate attempts to alter weight, the body would need to be better at putting a stop to weight loss, rather than gain. If we could lose weight just as easily as we gain it, people would drop dead with regularity, due to accidental starvation. That's not a winning strategy for the species, so we have not evolved that way. On the other hand, increased weight kills slowly, if at all, so the body is right to "prefer" that slow upward trend as a safety policy.

With regard to the studies above, during a severely limiting diet, rather than a body weight set point, it seems more likely to me that the body is focused on an *energetic* set point that it is in the habit of maintaining. The changes in hormone levels don't come from our body somehow weighing us, moment to moment. They come from signals related to nutrient availability. Glucose, amino acids, and break down products of fatty acids are all sensed in the hypothalamus (one of our most evolutionarily ancient brain regions). In addition, insulin levels inform the brain of how recently we have eaten.

Leptin and adiponectin are secreted from the fat cells and give a clear message regarding the long term storage of energy. CCK and PYY from the intestine let the hypothalamus know what's coming in the next few hours. Since one of the main roles of these hormones and regulators is to let us know whether or not to eat, it seems logical that they would react and adapt to coordinate greater appetite when we systematically eat less on a low-calorie diet.

*So with all this regulation working against our efforts to lose weight, how does anyone succeed?*

The fact is, very few people do succeed for any length of time. Apart from the very intense, semi-starvation diets designed to study the body's reaction to weight loss, the typical diet interventions reported in the medical literature show very modest one-year results. One of the landmark studies in weight loss and its effect on diabetes

15

risk highlights this well. The Diabetes Prevention Program was an extremely well-funded interventional study that sought to compare Metformin (a first line medicine for treating diabetes) to an intensive lifestyle program focusing on weight loss, better eating and exercise for diabetes prevention.

The encouraging finding, reported in 2002, was that you could reduce the 10 year risk of developing diabetes through a very intensive and prolonged effort with classes, group exercise, monitoring, and frequent follow up. Lifestyle worked even better than medication in this group. One of the reasons the study is so often cited is the fact that a very small overall weight loss, just 7% of body weight on average, reduced the risk of diabetes by 50%. From an obesity perspective, however, the fact that the average weight loss was 11.3 pounds (5.6 kg) in this very well-executed program is disheartening. I certainly wouldn't have had many of my weight management patients return for their second visit if I had promised them those results.

This study is not an outlier. In fact, the Diabetes Prevention Program results are better than most. In an analysis comparing the recommendations from Atkins, Zone, Ornish and the "LEARN" philosophies of weight loss, published in *JAMA* in 2007, researchers found one year weight loss to range from 4.8 pounds (2.2 kg) to 10.3 pounds (4.7 kg). I suppose I could mention where the different diets fell in that range, but really, who cares? My patients need to lose 100 pounds, not 10. And to be blunt, anyone who is trying to lose just 10 pounds, doesn't have a weight problem worthy of scientific scrutiny.

Commercial diets, when actually studied, do slightly worse than the trials run by physicians and professors. In a review of major commercial weight loss programs in the U.S., Adam Tsai and Thomas Wadden looked at Weight Watchers, Jenny Craig, L.A. Weight Loss, eDiets and meal replacement plans such as Optifast and Medifast. They found that one-year weight loss ranged from an *increase* of 3.2% body weight in one Weight Watchers group to a loss of 15% in a group counseling model with meal replacements at very low-calories. While the percentages are encouraging, (overall, about 7% weight loss at one year across all groups), the actual weight loss was quite modest across these studies, as the participants tended to be fairly light compared to physician-led trials. The Optifast meal replacement studies, which produced the greatest change in body weight, for example, averaged just 14 pounds (6.5 kg) lost at one year.

In my own clinic, I tracked results over three years for quality improvement purposes. I averaged the same results as most programs report: about 7% of total body weight for patients who stuck with me for more than 12 weeks. If I had included drop-outs (55%), the results would have looked far worse, as one must assume that the patients dropped out because my advice wasn't working for them. My patients were heavier than those in most studies, so that 7% equated to 27 pounds (12 kg) at an average of one year.

Since I had some patients who did remarkably well, I liked to look at my median weight loss, to get rid of the outlier effect (and really, we should insist on this for all weight loss studies). This was consistently running at 20 pounds (9 kg) through the years that I practiced weight loss medicine. 20 pounds may sound like an acceptable result for a clinic median if you fail to consider that the average weight for patients in my clinic was 305 pounds (137 kg) at first visit. So, a typical patient of mine could expect, through a tremendous amount of tracking, repeat visits, constant analyzing and continuing dietary change, to get from 305 to 285 pounds over the course of about a year.

Clinicians argue that a 5-10 percent change in body weight significantly improves risk factors such as blood sugar and triglycerides. This was the take home message from the Diabetes Prevention Program researchers. But whether doctors think the lab improvements that accompany a 10 or 20 pound loss are worth the effort may be irrelevant when we are specifically targeting obesity in a clinical, non-research setting. The more important question is: What do patients think about these numbers? This was tested by GD Foster and Thomas Wadden in 1997. As they reported in the *Journal of Consults in Clinical Psychology*, they examined patient expectations by asking new clients to their program to propose hard numbers for weight loss goals. Sixty women with average weight of 220 pounds (99 kg) were asked to define a one year goal that they would consider a "dream weight," a "happy weight," an "acceptable weight," or a "disappointed weight."

After a year, 47% of patient participants failed to reach even their "disappointed weight." This was despite the fact that the program was quite successful by medical standards, inducing, on average, a 35 pound (16 kg) weight loss.

In my weight loss practice, it was routine for new patients to express a desire to lose 100 pounds, or to reach a "normal" weight, despite the fact that this result almost never occurs. The reassurance that they would likely have improvements in their labs and reach a "not even disappointed" weight goal was something I discussed with hesitance. If obesity were a behavioral problem that could be reversed by an individual's effort, it wouldn't be unrealistic to shoot for a "dream weight." If what we weigh was under our personal control, we would be right to simply make a resolution, find a safe program and get going. We could put the blame on ourselves for being heavy and rightfully take charge of our weight by resolving to live differently. The unfortunate truth is that neither our current nor our future weight is under our control. Our internal regulatory mechanisms, responding to our food environment, decide our size and shape.

## References:

Bessesen DH, et. al. Trafficking of dietary fat and resistance to obesity. *Physiology and Behavior* 2008, 94(5): 59681-8.

Malhotra R, et. al. Young adult weight trajectories through midlife by body mass category. *Obesity* 2013, 21 (9): 1923-34.

Mozaffarian D, et. al. Changes in diet and lifestyle and long-term weight gain in women and men. *NEJM* 2011; 364: 2392-2404.

Leibel and Hirsch. Diminished energy requirements in reduced-obese patients. *Metabolism* 1984, 33(2): 164-170.

Rosenbaum, Hirsch, Gallagher, Leibel. Long-term persistence of adaptive thermogenesis in subjects who have maintained a reduced body weight. *American Journal of Clinical Nutrition* 2008, 88: 906-12.

Diabetes Prevention Program Research Group. Reduction in the incidence of type 2 diabetes with lifestyle intervention or metformin. *NEJM* 2002, 346: 393-403.

Leibel et. al. Changes in energy expenditure resulting from altered body weight. *NEJM* 1995, 332(10): 621-8.

www.NWCR.ws

Wyatt, HR, et. al. Resting energy expenditure in reduced-obese subjects in the National Weight Control Registry. *American Journal of Clinical Nutrition* 1999, 69: 1189-1193.

Sumathrin, et. al. Long-term persistence of hormonal adaptations to weight loss. *NEJM* 2011, 365: 1597-1604.

Tsai, AG and Wadden, TA. Systematic review: An evaluation of major commercial weight loss programs in the United States. *Annals of Internal Medicine* 2005, 142: 56-66.

Gardner, CD, et. al. Comparison of the Atkins, Zone, Ornish and LEARN diets for change in weight and related risk factors among overweight premenopausal women. *JAMA* 2007, 297(9): 969-77.

# Chapter 2

## Math, Time, and Obesity

You can discuss obesity and the science of weight regulation without using math . . . in the same way that you can discuss astronomy without using math. While there may be a way to present an argument in either field using just logic and pure reason, math becomes necessary as the questions become more complex and better defined. The mathematical regulation of body weight is easy to understand and comes directly from a simple energy balance equation with "R" denoting the amount of weight loss or gain, based on calories in, "I," minus calories expended, "E."

$R = I - E$

Of course, a person might feel that describing energy balance in this way is so obvious that it doesn't need to be discussed. This would be true, except that the "E" part of the equation is a little bit more complicated:

$E = DIT + PA + RMR + NEAT$

Because how we expend the calories we take in is broken down to four components: diet induced thermogenesis (DIT), which is the amount of energy we use digesting our food, plus physical activity (PA) like running, working-out, or any other purposeful movement, resting metabolic rate (RMR, which is the brain, heart, liver, and kidneys just keeping everything going) and "non-exercise activity thermogenesis," which we call NEAT (including fidgeting, posture and other movements not measurable as PA).

More importantly, all of these things are actually in constant flux. The above equations would really only suffice to describe the energy balance for a given moment in time. But we aren't much interested in math that describes how we are balanced at a particular moment. We want to know: What is the math that governs weight *change?* An equation to cover that question, at its absolute simplest, looks something like this:

$$E = ßI + mW + (1 - a)\{ciWpi - yi(A0+t/365)\} + r/1-r(DIT+PA+RMR) + C$$

Because we need calculus to describe how our bodies change over time. Don't worry, the equation above is just an example, and I don't thoroughly understand it either, but it demonstrates that each of the factors involved in energy expenditure, to describe weight loss or gain, would need modifiers that account for how they are regulated during periods of flux. So you would need to include a factor not just for the resting metabolism (RMR) but metabolism *as it fluctuates* daily with the change in weight and calories. Same idea for NEAT, PA, and DIT, until you end up with a much more complete and nuanced description, including the factors related to time.

The equations above are a small part of a larger construct elaborated by Diana Thomas in a 2009 paper that is part of a growing literature detailing mathematical attempts to model the human body's response to caloric imbalance. The math can be used to explain our population's weight gain in response to an overabundance of available calories, as well as how an individual body might react to an attempt to eat less or move more. It's complicated, but probably not something that we can gloss over if we want to truly understand what's happening with obesity.

## The 3500 Calorie Rule

Where all this becomes important is when we try to predict what's going to happen to a patient who decides to cut a certain number of calories per day in an effort to lose weight. There is a general recommendation given to overweight patients by most doctors and dietitians: Cut 500 calories per day and in one week, you will have skipped 3500 calories, which is the energy contained in one pound of fat. Using this formula, you should be able to lose a pound a week until you reach ideal body weight. The problem with the formula is that it simply doesn't work.

Yes, people lose weight when they cut calories, but they seem to need to cut much more than the magic 3500 calorie rule in the long run, and they tend to lose much more initially than the pound per week rule would predict. Weight loss is generally faster than expected initially and much slower after a month or so. One reason for the confusion is that the first week or two of weight loss is primarily a decrease in the amount of the food in the gut and changes in water balance. Those first 10 pounds aren't really pounds of fat.

More important is the fact that, even after we account for water shifting, losing weight grows gradually more difficult as time goes on. This has to do with a number of factors, but one that can be explained by mathematics is related to the body's composition changes during a weight loss regimen. We lose more body fat than lean mass. The body fat and the lean mass use different amounts of energy for maintenance, so the equation you use to predict how much a given calorie reduction will improve your body weight needs recalibration over time. As we get leaner, weight loss becomes slower and slower *on the same calories.*

The 3500 calorie rule only works well over a particular period of weeks, when a high proportion of the weight change is due to fat loss. From day 10 to about day 60 of a diet, the 3500 calorie rule works fine. As one becomes leaner, however, the new body composition re-sets the math, making weight loss harder and harder. This is just by the laws of physics, not by emotions or even the hormonal or metabolic changes known to occur. The graph of the weight loss over time is a curve, rather than a straight line. It's described by calculus, not algebra or arithmetic.

So, how do sophisticated mathematical models perform when applied to patient populations? Quite well. And getting better all the time. One of the main techniques used to build these models is to take data from well-done weight loss studies and use those numbers to create equations that will predict weight change in other populations. The proposed energy balance equations are based on observations of real human weight changes and as more studies are published, the models are re-tested and improved.

As in most scientific endeavors, the researchers at the top of this game are in friendly competition (I actually just assume this —perhaps it's very *unfriendly* competition. Maybe they are armed; I really couldn't say). To read the mathematical modeling articles published over the last several years is to watch the evolution of a new scientific tool: our ability to predict body weight changes accurately. Currently, the inputs are down to nine in the best model, developed by Kevin Hall and Carson Chow. The model parameters were published in a 2012 paper in *The Lancet*. An interactive, simplified, version of their model is available online at the NIDDK website.

### *The nine factors one can input into the online tool are:*

—Height

—Weight

—Age

—Sex

—Activity level (or metabolic rate, if known)

—Baseline calorie intake

—Percent of carbohydrate in the diet

—Grams of sodium in the diet

—Percent body fat (if known)

Using the first five, the program is able to estimate your current level of caloric intake and probable degree of body fat. You can estimate your percentage of carbohydrates and grams of sodium, or the program will assume you are near the U.S. average. Knowing your personal details can improve the predictions and playing with them on the website is one way to see how much each factor matters (spoiler: calories seem to be important).

The online tool is an easy way to get an understanding of the math, without any calculus. Don't be misled by the fact that sodium and percent carbohydrates are inputs into the model. Those are included for the sole purpose of getting the weight loss in the first week (which is based on changes in water, glycogen, and salt) correctly estimated. The model does not credit specific dietary choices, other than calories, as determining long term weight. Notice also that most inputs to the model are factors outside of one's control.

**Weight Loss Is Not Linear**

In the supplementary materials to the paper describing the Hall/Chow model, *Lancet* supplies readers with the mathematical discussion that would have been distracting in the main article. In the supplement, we are led to the master equation used for energy expenditure. Energy in, the "I" part of the equation, is just the calories we eat. That's never what's difficult to define. What's re-defined and clarified in the paper is the current best possible estimate of "E," which is our expenditure of energy. This master equation has too many Greek symbols for me to reproduce here, so I will try to convey the meaning of the equation in words:

Energy expenditure can be quantified as the sum of energy needed for resting metabolism added to the amount of energy needed to digest food and move the body. The amount of energy needed to do these things varies by overall body weight, percent body fat, age, and sex. The amount of carbohydrate and salt in the diet can alter weight, particularly in the short term, through changes in glycogen and water balance. Attempts to change the energy balance by altering intake of food will produce variable results depending upon weight and body composition. Since the energy used to create fat and lean tissue, the energy needed to maintain these different tissues, and the energy those tissues make available to the rest of the body during a reducing regimen, are all different, the rate of weight change will vary depending upon the ratio of fat to lean tissue. When the ratio of fat to lean tissue is altered, in either direction, the predicted weight loss or gain that results from the energy balance equation will change in response. An individual's ability to partition energy to the different tissues, regulate movement of macronutrients and maintain nutrient balance will account for intra-individual variations in weight loss.

*Maybe I should have just written the equation . . .*

While the above paragraph may not be clearest in this book, it does give one a sense of the multitude of factors addressed by the math model. Each of the sentences above represents one of the variables in the researchers' equation. When a patient asks me a simple question about how much they need to eat, or how much they would need to cut to reach a certain goal, I reflect on the true complexity that exists in the body's accounting of the "ins and outs" of energy balance. Since the mathematicians are in competition to create the most complete description while keeping the equation parsimonious, we can assume that there are no unnecessary inputs. All of these inputs come from established science that can't be argued with, but the mathematical outcomes described by the Hall/Chow equation may be more precise than previous models and the ramifications are surprising.

Weight loss does reach a plateau, but that plateau is not in the typical 6-8 months seen in most diet studies. The calculations demonstrate that a given caloric intervention does not run linearly at a pound or two per week, but curves gradually toward its goal and will yield only about half the weight loss in the first year. It will take two more years to reach the point where the slope of the line documenting the weight loss curve will appear totally horizontal and no more weight loss is possible. This eventual plateau will represent the new energy balance at the new weight, given a new fat/lean ratio for the individual. At that point, the individual can be said to be in thermodynamic stability, with a new "I" and new "E" that represent a truly different metabolic state.

In the example below, I simulated myself, using the Hall/Chow model, beginning at 145 pounds and reducing my daily diet from 2500 calories to 2000 calories per day. Note the different results predicted using the 3500 rule vs. the calculus model:

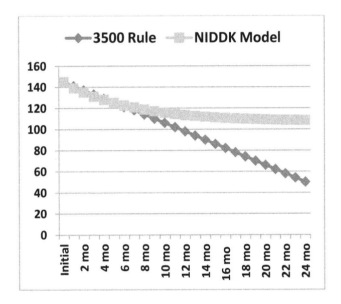

Both equations predict that I will quickly reach an unhealthy weight, but the NIDDK simulator shows my body adjusting to a near horizontal equilibrium in the second year, whereas the 3500 rule shows me attaining my 3rd grade weight of 50 pounds, or likely dropping dead somewhere along the way . . . *on 2000 calories per day.* Surely there is something wrong with that math.

Now let's look at a perhaps more reasonable example. Take my average clinic patient, a 305-pound (139 kg) 55-year-old female. Baseline calorie intake for an office worker who doesn't exercise, is 3000 per day. A reduction to 2000 cal/day produces the following:

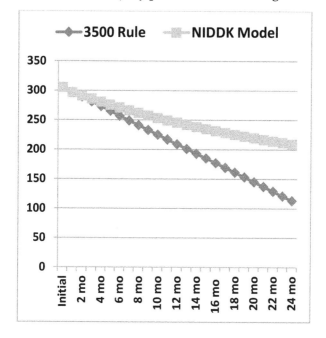

This calculated plot of weight loss over a two year period shows a model simulated loss of 96 pounds, assuming strict adherence to a 2000 calorie diet. The 3500 calorie rule again produces a highly exaggerated trajectory. In this case, a 192-pound weight loss resulting in a final weight of 113 pounds. This is a result that I've never seen in the clinic, nor has it been reported in any diet study, not even from bariatric surgery. So these two examples give us a sense of how well a more complex math-based model, utilizing calculus, compares to standard dietary recommendations and the 3500 calorie rule. At this point, we can dispense with the 3500 calorie rule as too inaccurate.

Note that the NIDDK model shows that an individual cutting 500-1000 calories per day, would still, on day 730, be in active weight loss mode, not yet in need of reducing calories further to continue weight loss. One of the inescapable mathematical truths I discovered with patients, which also manifests in the math models, is that very heavy patients, such as anyone over 300 pounds, should be able to lose weight for at least two years on 2000 calories per day.

### The Diet Does Not "Stop Working"

My experience, working in a day-to-day medical practice, was that very few individuals are able to stay on a dietary intervention long enough to test these models. When we look at any given group, most people will fall off of a diet because they are hungry, or don't like the new rules, or suffer an illness. In other words, "life" gets in the way of eating like a robot that can be predicted by math models. This is not the fault of the dieting individual; it is simply the human body regulating food intake to match its needs. While some exceptional individuals may be able to keep a rigid diet for years on end, it is much more common for weight to rebound. In any large group, the number of individuals who will experience weight rebound is far larger than the number who will keep weight off permanently. For this reason, neither of the above example weight loss trajectories have ever been seen as an average for an entire group of people trying to lose weight. Published studies of weight loss trials show a plot of the group that invariably looks something like this:

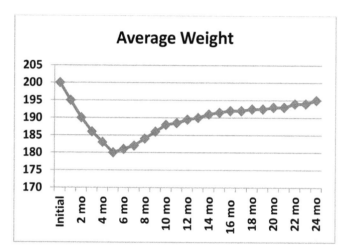

Whether it's a trial of a weight loss medication or a new diet philosophy, the average weight loss will always follow the above pattern. Initial weight loss abruptly reverses direction sometime around 6 months, with a gradual return to the pre-intervention weight over a year or two. One cannot help but wonder: What happens at six months?

When reading an article in a medical journal, the answer to that question can usually found in the "methods" section of the paper, which describes that the participants attended biweekly sessions for six months, or received meal replacements for six months, or medication for six months . . . with the inevitable consequence that as soon as the intervention is scaled back to see what naturally results, the return to baseline starts fairly immediately.

Generally, to get a study published, you need to follow the participants for one to two years total. But this is much too long to keep the majority of participants engaged, so after the initial six month intensive study period, the weigh-ins and contact are generally relaxed to 3 month intervals as the study winds down and collects data. At this point, the main intervention has ceased, and the researcher want to know what the longer term effect of the six month trial will be. The interventions carried out for studies tend to be expensive and time consuming, so a stopping point is necessary for practical reasons. This six month turning point is arbitrary; the graph of weight loss and regain looks the same in three month trials, but the upswing just starts sooner. The graph has the same shape for bariatric surgery studies; the trend is just much steeper and deeper on the downside. Regardless of how well the intervention works, the loss will always reverse itself in the long run for the average individual.

Working backward from this highly reproducible graph of study results to the calorie numbers that would be required to produce it, Carson Chow and Kevin Hall, in a 2014 article published in *Physiology and Behavior,* show that this pattern comes from patients, on average, returning *completely* to their baseline diet within the first year. It can take several more months for that relative increase in calories to fully work into the body as stored fat and increased weight. The full weight re-gain lags the full resumption of higher calorie consumption by several months because weight change happens on a calculus-based time curve. The results of a given dietary intervention are simply much slower than we generally realize. This holds true both on the way down and on the way up. What does this mean for dieting? It means that *almost no one has tried anything long enough to know if it works.* You would have to continue whatever you are doing for years before deciding whether it was the right diet for you.

Think about how a diet goes: If one adheres to the new food rules perfectly (which is the exception, not the rule) the initial weight loss goes fairly smoothly. If one starts to gradually relax the rules, one is still, on average, calorie negative day-to-day, so the weight loss continues. After a weekend binge, for example, one might actually weigh five or six pounds more, but that's the weight of the food and salt and water, not actual new fat accumulation. A few days of following the rules and things will seem alright on the scale again. As one "cheats" off and on, for a good deal of time, the body is (again, averaging over a few days) in negative caloric balance and still continues to lose. At this point, the dieting individual has no idea what works or doesn't work, decides to abandon the whole project, and just resume customary eating. However, the body doesn't return to the pre-diet weight for *one or two more years,* teaching the individual . . . what? Perhaps that the amount of food isn't the problem and that weight gain or loss must be due to something else. What other conclusion could a reasonable person draw after having such strange results from a dietary intervention? Do this a few times throughout your adult life and you might start to doubt the truth of what a calorie is.

**A Calorie Is a Calorie. So What?**

What is a calorie anyway? The term is actually a misnomer, since when we say "calorie" we actually mean "kilocalorie," as in, one thousand calories. But by convention, the two terms are interchangeable and what is referred to is the amount of energy required to raise the temperature of one cubic centimeter of water by one degree centigrade. Calories in food can be calculated in a lab using a device not surprisingly called a calorimeter, which essentially burns the food to see how much heat is produced. This is then assigned a calorie value which represents that heat energy. In our body, calories are measured . . . absolutely nowhere. Calories don't exist in the body. We have no calorimeter and we don't "burn" anything at all. What we do is utilize nutrients: fat, protein and carbohydrate molecules, in various ways. Some of the energy stored in the bonds of these molecules is released in chemical reactions to make the body's universal energy currency: ATP.

ATP is to the body what the "calorie" is to the lab. ATP is a generic form of temporary stored energy that facilitates most of the reactions within cells by giving up a highly charged group to trade with other molecules that need that charge. It takes energy to add a phosphate group onto "Adenosine Di-Phosphate" (ADP) to make it "Adenosine Tri-Phosphate" (ATP). That energy comes from the food we eat. When that third phosphate leaves the molecule again (when highly charged ATP goes back to being plain old ADP) it releases the energy that was holding the third phosphate to the molecule. Nearby molecules use that energy to do biochemical work on themselves and neighboring molecules, such as breaking them in two, coupling them together, forming chains, or changing their shape. Molecular reactions, not fires, are what use up energy in the body. The end products are the same: carbon dioxide, water and heat. But the variable pathways required to create ATP in a body have inefficiencies that make it impossible to state with any certainty how many lab measured calories will yield a certain amount of ATP in our cells. Even if we could write an equation that translated calories to molecules of ATP, the main factor controlling weight wouldn't be the equation describing "in" and "out," but what happens to the energy as it's converted, mobilized, and distributed in a living animal.

In a 2004 review entitled "Thermodynamics of Weight Loss Diets," Eugene Fine and Richard Feinman argued that changes in *what* we eat, specifically the balance of protein to the other nutrients, can affect the amount of ATP produced from our food. Rather than argue which nutrients are more filling and cause us to stop eating sooner (which is the logic fueling many weight loss recommendations), the authors review how each macronutrient is processed and how efficiently each can be expected to create ATP for cellular energy. They point out that the body has various inefficiencies for energy production based on the amount of energy needed to produce the usable forms of the food molecules, transport nutrients through the body, generate body heat, create complex structural components and break them back down. All of these decrease the yield of energy one would expect from measuring calories in the lab. From glucose, our production is shown to be 38.5% efficient, for example. This means that more energy is lost in making the energy (as heat, $CO_2$ and $H_2O$) than is produced in ATP. This is a theoretical average based upon the known biochemistry, not something that scientists have measured. In theory, individual variability in these biochemical processes would explain why some of us run fast and lean and others run slow and heavy.

The authors go on to elaborate an idea that provokes controversy, which is that the different macronutrients vary in their ability to produce energy. They show that the most ATP can be produced from directly using fat in the diet, then glucose, then protein, with 40.9%, 38.5% and 33% efficiency ratings. All three yield less energy when they go through intermediate steps for storage, such as when we try to get the ATP energy back out of stored glycogen in the liver, fatty acids from the fat cells, or amino acids from the muscles. Again, variability in storage and mobilization of these molecules could account for much of the observed human variation in metabolism. The most *inefficient* pathway would be to eat protein, build new muscle, and then break it down again to create ATP. That path is shown to be only 27% efficient. Note that these numbers have nothing to do with DIT, NEAT, PA discussed above. They are variables within the body, within the resting metabolism that the authors argue can possibly be altered by dietary choice. Since RMR is the largest component of how much energy we use (60%), and the different macronutrients produce different effects on RMR, the implication is that *what* we eat, not just *how much,* is an important target for weight loss strategies. While this work is theoretical, and has not been tested in terms of any practical applications, it raises possibilities that deserve attention. The next two chapters deal with questions regarding *what* we eat in more detail.

## References:

Thomas, DM, et. al. A mathematical model of weight change with adaptation. *Math, Biosciences and Engineering* 2009, 6(4): 873-887.

Hall, KD, et. al. Quantification of the effect of energy imbalance on bodyweight. *Lancet* 2011, 378 (9793): 826-37.

Chow, CC and Hall, KD. The dynamics of human body weight change. *PLOS Computational Biology* 2008, 4(3): e1000045.

Chow, CC and Hall, KD. Short and long term energy intake patterns and their implications for human body weight regulation. *Physiology and Behavior* 2014, 134: 60-65.

Fine, EJ and Feinman, RD. Thermodynamics of weight loss diets. *Nutrition and Metabolism* 2004, 1(15).

# Chapter 3

# The Carbohydrate Hypothesis

Any discussion of carbohydrates in the diet must deal with the Atkins conception of weight loss, because it is so commonly used, and it rests in the middle of the debate regarding the causes of weight gain. Anyone trying to figure out why we've become obese needs to decide, at some point, whether Atkins had the cause and effect of obesity and diabetes correct.

It's easy to dismiss Dr. Atkins. His books are self-promoting (he named the diet, which pre-existed him by 150 years, after himself) and full of hyperbole:

*"Atkins is the most successful weight loss - and weight maintenance - program of the last quarter of the twentieth century. The fact is, by methods you're about to learn, it works an astonishing proportion of the time for the vast majority of men and women." —Dr. Atkins' New Diet Revolution, 2002.*

He frequently referenced the medical literature obliquely, or added references after bold pronouncements that correspond to papers that don't actually support his point. He invented words like "vitanutrients." He published weight loss books with his name in bold letters, but no peer-reviewed studies of his outcomes. He made sweeping generalizations about the effects of dietary choices without any real attempt to validate his ideas using the scientific rigor necessary to publish in journals. His books sometimes get the science just plain wrong, such as when he contends that insulin is a glucose transporter. He was wrong about a lot of things, but as a friend of mine used to apply to me, "even a blind squirrel occasionally finds a nut." We shouldn't confuse the objections we have with Dr. Atkins's style, or even his reasoning, with objections to his advice. We should look at his proposition, if we can, without bias. The components of the carbohydrate hypothesis are:

—Carbohydrates (sugar, breads, pastas, fruit, soda) raise insulin levels

—Insulin's job is to move sugar and fat out of the blood

—It does this mainly by opening up fat cells for storage

—It also decreases fat break down

—Increased insulin means increased storage and less fat burning

Therefore:

—High sugar causes high insulin causes obesity

This mechanism is, in fact, an accurate description of how energy gets shuttled into cells. But to show that sugar and other carbohydrates *uniquely* fatten us, we need to consider whether the system above, which operates in lean individuals as well, has somehow been driven to excess by our changing diet.

To critically review what macronutrient choice does for our struggle with obesity, we can do no better than discuss the work of Gary Taubes. I know many doctors who disagree with what Gary Taubes has concluded about obesity, but none who have actually read his book. To finish *Good Calories, Bad Calories* (his 2007 encyclopedic history of the low-fat diet hypothesis and why it is false —more aptly titled for the UK printing as *The Diet Delusion*) is to be convinced that we have been pre-ordained to become heavier by the bad advice that has come to us from the USDA and the American Heart Association. He makes the best case I've seen that we are increasingly overweight and obese because we eat too much carbohydrate. The book walks us through the history of low-fat dieting, how the common wisdom that eating fat causes weight gain *became* the common wisdom and why it has inadvertently backfired. He provides exhaustive evidence to back up his story: He documents hundreds of interviews with the scientists who have written the guidelines and position statements that inform our judgment of what constitutes a healthy diet. He also lays out the findings of hundreds of peer-reviewed research trials and analyses that lead directly to his conclusion that Dr. Atkins actually stumbled across the truth. Taubes shows that the low-fat advice that dominated the popular awareness for 40 years was an accident of which experts happened to be in power in research circles at a certain period of our history.

That some of our best scientists believed that a low-fat diet would give us better health and longevity is without question. But those scientists, Taubes argues quite convincingly, were simply wrong. In addition, they were frequently misunderstood, misquoted and used to push an agenda. They had some decent, but incomplete, evidence about the causes of heart disease that was taken as gospel by government agencies and medical reporters that needed something clear to tell the public. The best way to eat to avoid heart disease was taken as the best way to eat, period. In reality, the evidence was never even clear regarding fat and heart disease. The data had nuances that couldn't be fit into a headline and two generations of us gained a lot of weight trying to avoid "getting fat" by avoiding eating fat. As evidence grew that avoiding dietary fat was not a cure or a preventive strategy for obesity or heart disease, the message went unheard, because it was inconvenient and hard to understand. In fact, though, eating fat doesn't "make you fat" any more than eating cholesterol gives you high cholesterol, or eating salt gives you a high salt level in the blood (or high blood pressure, for most of us). These points are all evaluated and dismissed in the book. But more importantly, Taubes presents the case that the heart-focused eating that prevailed from 1970 to 2000, had an unexpected side effect: the obesity epidemic.

The argument in *Good Calories, Bad Calories* is straightforward: Because we were told to avoid high-fat foods, we looked for labels and products that claimed to be "low-fat." The packaged food industry, in order to produce the highly enjoyable taste experience we've come to expect from anything that comes in a wrapper, had to replace the fat with something we'd enjoy. That something was carbohydrates, the complex kind and the simple kind, such as sucrose and fructose. Coming at a time when we finally had enough disposable income to eat pre-packaged food every day of the week, we essentially snacked, drove-through, and micro-waved ourselves into our current state of obesity by letting the food companies feed us tasty carbohydrate treats.

None of this is hard to believe and really wouldn't bother most doctors. What's more challenging to accept is Taubes's argument that calories simply don't matter when it comes to weight gain. They mediate the process, but excess calorie consumption is considered an accident of too much carbohydrate consumption, not the underlying cause of obesity. Sugars and carbs are viewed as essential to the process, or even considered almost a "toxin" when it comes to our metabolism.

His other controversial stance is that dietary fat doesn't matter. It doesn't cause obesity and in fact, eating it (at least the right kinds) will help you avoid a heart attack while losing weight. Does this make any sense? The evidence is mounting in his favor. Taubes is certainly right that we need to remember that the body isn't an empty set of tubes and circuits that utilizes fuels only in the forms they are ingested. The human organism is a complex array of chemical reactions, hormonal signaling, energy balancing and nutrient sensing that acts on the cellular and molecular level to produce health. Food is converted by a host of processes in the organism after ingestion. All of these processes are regulated by an array of genes and hormones that have evolved over millennia, perhaps demonstrating that we've been through these fluctuations before. Lately, the regulation of our weight seems to be off-kilter, causing a perhaps unprecedented weight gain in many populations. The question for the moment is: How much of the regulation of weight gain is driven by carbohydrate in the diet?

The carbohydrate hypothesis begins with the assertion that we are currently eating more carbohydrate than we were a few decades ago. By various measures, including USDA numbers of what gets produced by the food industry and surveys of how people typically eat on a day-to-day basis, it's been shown that we've had a reasonably large shift in our consumption patterns. In a recent paper looking at the percentage of carbohydrates, fat and protein in the U.S. diet between the early 1970's and 2006, Austin and colleagues report that carbohydrates, as a percentage of diet, have increased over those 30 years. The researchers chose to utilize the data from NHANES, which relies upon self-report. By this method of measurement, carbohydrate percentage is rising. This has happened while the percentages of protein and fat have decreased and the obesity rate in the country has tripled:

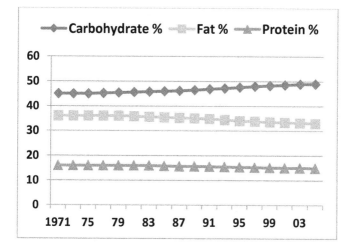

Since obesity rates have risen markedly in sync with the increase in carbohydrates and decrease in fat, the carbohydrate hypothesis argues that the USDA, your cardiologist and the well-meaning folks who make "low-fat" sour cream potato chips have caused us to make a huge mistake: while avoiding fat for the last 30 years, we have substituted carbohydrates. The obesity and type 2 diabetes epidemics are the result.

But do these data really support that view? Looking at the numbers, between the periods 1971-75 and 2005-06, everyone in the U.S. seems to have learned to eat more. Separated into groups considered normal weight, overweight and obese, the average person in each group ate about 200 more calories per day. Meanwhile, the percentage of carbohydrate increased from 45% to 49% while fat decreased 36% to 33% and protein decreased from 16% to 15%. So you could certainly choose to draw the conclusion, looking at the graph above, that American adults are susceptible to public health messaging and that they reduced their fat consumption during this 30 year period. That would be a mistake:

| Wt. | Norm (70s) | Over (70s) | Obese (70s) | Norm (05) | Over (05) | Obese (05) |
|---|---|---|---|---|---|---|
| Pro | 101g | 101g | 104g | 108g | 100g | 104g |
| Fat | 105g | 98g | 99g | 104g | 95g | 100g |
| Carb | 274g | 254g | 244g | 334 | 311 | 308 |
| Cals | 2551 | 2416 | 2348 | 2798 | 2581 | 2608 |
| Cal. Diff | | | | +247 | +165 | +229 |

What this table of the amounts of food eaten demonstrates is that we are eating the same *total quantity* of protein and fat, by grams, as we've always eaten. The only thing that's changed between the seventies and now is that we've added, on average, 50 grams, or about 200 more calories' worth, of carbs. Not substituted, but *added*. The entire increase in calories in our daily consumption over the last 30 years is due to carbohydrate. We haven't heeded any public health advice about avoiding fat; we are eating all the fat we ever did, we've just increased carbs (and the calories they supply) on top of that.

Why are we all heavier? If these numbers are to be believed, the obese folks have increased their intake, on average, 229 cals per day. This would translate to 81,760 excess calories per year, which (if each pound of fat is produced by approximately 3500 excess cals consumed) would yield a weight gain of 23 pounds. That seems pretty close to the reported increase in weight of obese people over the last three decades, which is 18 pounds on average. The only problem is that the calories resulting in that 23 pounds of weight gain would be *per year*. That's right, if these numbers are accurate, the average obese person would have gained *700 pounds* between the two NHANES surveys. Since normal weight respondents in the data-set report eating 247 calories more daily, they'd be 750 pounds heavier . . .

Here is where we, again, run into the limits of using the 3500 calorie = a pound rule. As you get heavier, you expend and take in more calories to sustain your mass, so the increase becomes less excessive as a new equilibrium is found. Plugging the increase of 229 calories into the NIDDK bodyweight simulator (discussed last chapter), we find that the expected weight gain, depending upon starting assumptions, would be close to 20 pounds. That's quite a bit different from 750 pounds, nearly identical to the 18 pounds reported, and demonstrates why calculus is needed in these discussions, rather than simple arithmetic.

Notice that this study confirms (by the self-report of many thousands of individuals) what Dr. Liebel measured in the study we discussed in Chapter One. "The obese and control subjects required comparable caloric intakes." While the obese group reports an increase of 229 calories more over the three decades, the lean participants report eating 247 calories more, which is an indistinguishable difference, given the known difficulties in assessing caloric intake with precision. While we have reason to believe that individuals under-report calories they eat, we have little reason to suspect that they all systematically report these changes in macronutrient composition. Since the lean and overweight report eating the same macronutrient ratio as the obese, we can posit that we are all exposed to the same food environment and eat roughly the same, but some of us are resistant while others are susceptible to weight gain.

Our increased obesity correlates to an increase in the amount of calories eaten, composed entirely of carbohydrate, and this has happened during a period when carbohydrate has measurably increased as a percentage of diet. But does this mean that carbohydrate is somehow "bad" for us? The question remains: Is it the carbs, or the calories they supply, that ultimately cause obesity?

**Are All Calories Equal?**

If carbohydrates are somehow more "fattening" than the other macronutrients, reducing carbohydrates during weight loss should show signs of improving other internal regulatory factors, in addition to weight. Cara Ebbeling and colleagues looked at this question by putting volunteers on equal calorie diets for three months. In a 2012 study reported in *JAMA*, the researchers followed 21 volunteers on variable carbohydrate diets and assessed their hormonal and metabolic responses. The question they were asking was whether there was a "metabolic advantage" of a low-carbohydrate diet, as argued by Atkins and many professionals who see weight loss clients. After losing, on average, 12.5% of body weight over 12 weeks, the subjects were stabilized over the following month, to find the calorie amount each needed to maintain that loss. After the stabilization period, each subject served as his own control, observing a high carb, medium carb, and low-carb diet for four weeks at a time. All the diets were of equal calories, intended to maintain the stable weight, so the only difference was the *composition* of the diets.

What they found was that there was, indeed, evidence that carbohydrate restriction worked better than other strategies. The known response of our body to reduced calories is to reduce metabolic rate. This response occurred in all the volunteers, on all the diets, but it was blunted in the low-carb group. Instead of decreasing resting energy expenditure by 205 cals/day (as the high carb/low-fat group did), the low-carb group decreased by only 138. Total energy expenditure (which includes activity and energy spent digesting food) was decreased by 423 cals/day in the high carb group vs. 97 cals per day in the low-carb group. That's a pretty significant difference. If this finding could be reproduced in a larger study sample, the ramifications for dieting would be enormous. Who wouldn't rather eat the 236 calorie difference in efficiency between the two diets?

If the low-carbohydrate approach has a metabolic advantage, what would be the internal mechanism? The most often proposed mechanism, from Atkins in 1971 to the present day, is the concept of turning on "ketosis." This often misunderstood term refers to a state of measurable use of fat for fuel in the body. It is often confused, by laypersons and doctors alike, with "ketoacidosis" which is a dangerous state encountered by some type 1 diabetic patients with severely low insulin levels. Ketosis, on the other hand, refers simply to the presence of "ketones" in the body at a high enough level that they can be measured in the blood or urine. Ketones are a normal breakdown product of fat metabolism and have a constant presence in our moment-to-moment energy balance.

We naturally produce some ketones at all times, especially while we sleep, but at a very low level in most people. The role of ketones throughout a normal day is to provide energy when glucose is low. So, if there is a long period between meals, or when an individual is sleeping, the body uses fat energy, in the form of ketones, to keep cellular metabolism running smoothly. Getting a large amount of ketones in the blood happens in one of two ways: fasting, or severe carbohydrate restriction. Fasting, of course, is simply the act of severely restricting fat and protein along with the carbs, so the distinction is not terribly important. Without carbohydrate, we break down fat to ketones and other smaller molecules to supply energy to the body, with the brain first on the list. If your insulin system is still active, your body has no problem with the switch of fuels. Why low-carbohydrate advocates believe that ketosis is necessary for "true" weight loss is likely because ketones come from fat breakdown, so it's considered evidence that stored fat is being burned, rather than fat that's been eaten, or mobilized from the liver or other tissues. This is probably not true and also neglects the fact that lipids, in the form of triglycerides and free fatty acids, are circulating through the body all day long. The measured ketones while dieting could easily be from your last meal, particularly when one is following the high fat recommendation of Atkins. Fatty chains of shorter lengths float through the fluid of all of our cells, right next to the mitochondria, converting to ketone body intermediates when being used as fuel in alternation with glucose. There is no real need to "unlock" the particular fat molecules that reside in adipose tissue. The ketones are in our cells all the time and are a normal balancing force in daily metabolism.

The main selling point of the Atkins diet and to a lesser extent "paleo" and other low-carb diets, is that you can still eat plenty of protein and fat and maintain ketosis. This allows you to avoid hunger, by "eating as much as you want," while still losing weight. While this is in some sense true, "as much as you want" when you can't include any carbohydrate is invariably *many fewer calories* than one would typically eat. Since carbohydrates make up 50-55% of daily calories, critics point out that eliminating half of our normal food options is bound to make anyone lose weight. You simply can't find enough protein and fat to make up the difference. Most "convenience" foods, including anything in a wrapper that one can grab on the go, are carbohydrate-based. Protein, fat and vegetables require planning, cooking, and preparation each day. The planning, cooking, and preparation would likely have a beneficial effect on anyone's diet, regardless of the specific recommendation. My own experiments trying to "do Atkins" have been disrupted by the fact that even most flavors of beef jerky are too high in carbohydrates to fit the recommendations. It can be safely said that there are many fewer opportunities to eat when one eliminates carbohydrate and one is often faced with a choice between breaking the diet rules, or skipping a meal altogether.

**What Is Lost When We Lose Weight?**

At least as far back as 1976, researchers have been looking at the relative advantage of diets which promote ketosis. This was before the "obesity crisis" was conceptualized and before any noticeable shifts in macronutrients had occurred in the food supply. In the *Journal of Clinical Investigation*, Yang and Van Itallie subjected six "grossly obese male subjects" to three diets, each lasting 10 days. The diets were: complete starvation (just non-caloric fluids), an 800 calorie ketogenic diet, and an 800 calorie mixed diet. These diets were given to each volunteer alternating with more relaxed periods of 1200 calorie diets. In this way, each participant served as his own control, enabling the researchers to account for the variability that exists in various individuals' biological response to diet manipulations. The different diets were:

—Ketogenic diet: 25% protein, 70% fat and 5% carbohydrate

—Mixed diet: 25% protein, 30% fat and 45% carbohydrate

—Fasting: 0% protein, 0% fat and 0% carbohydrate

—1200 cal diet: 17% protein, 30% fat and 53% carbohydrate (considered typical in 1976)

They alternated these diets in the subjects, using the 1200 calorie diets as a sort of wash-out process between the ten-day study periods. The question they were trying to answer was: Does diet composition make a difference in weight loss? They were also curious to study *what* exactly was lost: fat, lean tissue, or water. Each subject lived in the hospital for 50 days, alternating the diets while getting weighed daily, and allowing all of his urine and feces to be collected for analysis.

The researchers estimated calories burned in activity by having the subjects keep logs of all of their activities and by estimating the caloric burn by indirect calorimetry. This involves breathing into a tube which analyzes how much oxygen you are consuming in different situations. If you're sitting still, you burn a certain amount of oxygen and this can be measured in the air you inhale versus the air you exhale. If you're running on a treadmill, naturally, you use up more oxygen than when sitting still and that is reflected in the air collected in the tube as an increase in the carbon dioxide level. This translates pretty well to how much energy your body is using during different activities. The researchers recorded how many hours each volunteer spent performing various daily activities to estimate how many calories each were burning.

Today, if you wanted to look at body composition, you'd use a dexa scanner (the same machine we use for bone density scans). Dexa is quick, easy, and accurate for distinguishing lean mass from fat mass. In the seventies, they did some mathematical gymnastics involving nitrogen that I won't describe here, mostly because I don't understand them at all. However, by their description, it is clear they were able to use the nitrogen balance to estimate whether muscle mass, protein balance or fat balance was changing in these subjects who lost weight. What did they find?

The starvation periods produced the most weight loss, followed by the 800 calorie ketogenic diet and then, the 800 calorie balanced diet. The subjects lost, on average, 750 grams (1.7 pounds) per day while fasting, 466 grams (1.0 pound) per day on the ketogenic diet and 277 grams (0.6 pounds) on the balanced, or mixed, diet as they call it.

What does this mean? Of course, fasting causes the most weight loss and it's an excellent method for slimming down, but of limited utility in the long run. Between the other two diets, low-carb vs. balanced, does the low-carb diet really produce almost *double* the weight loss? 0.6 vs. 1.0 pound per day? Actually, no. What this study showed, very clearly by 1976 scientific standards, is that low-carb diets are, in the short term at least, *dehydrating*.

When they measured *what* was lost on the 800 calorie diets, they found that both the low-carb ketogenic and the balanced diet, produced the same amount of fat loss, the same amount of muscle loss, but very different amounts of water loss. The balanced diet caused an average of 102 grams (0.2 pounds) of water loss while the ketogenic diet caused 284 grams (0.6 pounds) of water loss, daily. This accounts for the entire difference in lost weight.

One conclusion we might draw from this is that a mixed, or balanced, diet that reduces calories, will cause a reliable, slow weight loss and you can count on doubling that by eating the same calories without any carbohydrates. This doubling will come entirely from water loss, rather than actual fat cells giving up their contents. This study shows that the low-carb approach works as well as another diet and gives encouraging results on the scale (which may be important for patient adherence). But the study does, perhaps, suggest an explanation for how reversible our quick low-carb weight loss can be: if half the weight we lose in the beginning is actually just water, we are always just a couple of meals away from putting five pounds back on. The carbs, salt and the liquids that we use to wash down a restaurant meal will make us feel as if one night, or a weekend, of indulgence has reversed all of our gains, simply because water weight fluctuates so dramatically. I believe that a lot of the enthusiasm that low-carb diets provoke and the following frustration they cause, is in fact due to these water shifts, which exaggerate our observations in both directions, at least in the initial phase of low-carb dieting.

**Critical Evaluation of Low-Carb Diets**

The first longer term, randomized controlled trial of the specific low-carbohydrate approach advocated by Atkins was published in the *New England Journal* in 2003. One of the authors, James O. Hill, had given a talk that same year in Washington DC that I'd attended. In response to the question of what were "three take-away points to remember for obesity treatment," Dr. Hill spontaneously responded that he could only think of two: portion control and pedometers. I thought that was a great answer (from his perspective), and I think it qualifies him as an unbiased examiner of the low-carbohydrate hypothesis. In the study, the researchers compared weight loss and cardiac risk factors in a group of 63 participants at 3, 6 and 12 months. Half of the volunteers followed the Atkins low-carb/high protein/high fat approach and the others followed a traditional low-fat recommendation. What they found was that the weight loss was indeed greater for the low-carb group for the first six months (7 kg vs. 3.2kg), but the difference disappeared at the one year mark. With regard to cardiac risk, the low-carbohydrate diet was superior to low-fat. This perhaps suggests the obvious: Atkins is superior, but harder to maintain than more "reasonable" diet recommendations.

In a 2007 *American Journal of Clinical Nutrition* comprehensive review of low-carbohydrate outcomes, Eric Westman (who is frequently quoted by Dr. Atkins in his books) and colleagues collected results from randomized controlled diet studies comparing low-carbohydrate to usual weight loss recommendations. Their tabulated results of six well-performed, decently large, studies show a consistent advantage of low-carb over low-fat diets: 9.3 kg (20.5 pounds) vs. 4.5 kg (9.9 pounds) over periods of time ranging 3 months to one year. These studies were long enough and used modern methods to show that the difference was not due to temporary water losses. However, within individual studies, some of the differences between the weight loss outcomes were insignificant, so that those studies, taken alone, would not support the argument that low-carbohydrate diets are superior. The authors show that cardiac risk factors were either unchanged (cholesterol) or improved (triglycerides) using the low-carbohydrate methods. The authors suggest, in a more scientifically rational and reserved tone than Atkins used, that there is no reason to fear low-carb methods and a there is good reason to use it as the first line of defense for obesity and diabetes. It can be safely said that this group contains low-carbohydrate advocates (Volek and Phinney wrote the 2010 update of the Atkins diet revolution book), but they advocate it from a more scientifically sound platform.

Notice that we keep stumbling across the finding (from 1976 to the present) that low-carb diets produce about twice as much weight loss as low-fat diets. The vast majority of studies looking at this question have found either that, or that there was no difference between diets. The science supporting the low-carb hypothesis and the proposed solution has good internal consistency: Eating carbohydrate *does* raise blood sugar more than eating protein or fat. It *does* raise insulin more than the other macronutrients (protein raises insulin about 1/2 as much, fat almost negligibly). Insulin *does* increase storage of energy and turn off fat breakdown. Insulin, when taken as a medicine, *almost invariably* causes weight gain. Furthermore, eating fewer carbohydrates *does* lower blood sugar and insulin. Low-carb dieting is arguably more effective for weight loss. Given all this, we must ask: Why do so many very good scientists reject the carbohydrate hypothesis of obesity causation?

The carbohydrate hypothesis is a coherent description of fat cell energy regulation and it may be the simplest explanation we can use to understand how we gain weight. However, it only remains coherent through a fair amount of simplification of the regulatory pathways. Nothing said about the actions of insulin is inaccurate in the "carbs cause obesity" thinking, but the focus on insulin *alone* may be misguided. In addition to being one of many hormones involved in energy regulation, insulin has a variety of actions in our body, not necessarily related to weight homeostasis. A baseline level of insulin is secreted into the blood by the beta cells of the pancreas at all times. When insulin is low, as during our overnight fast, the liver maintains our blood sugar level through a process called "gluconeogenesis." When we eat, the pancreas responds by releasing more insulin over the course of the following two hours. Higher insulin turns off gluconeogenesis in the liver. It also manages the incoming sugar energy from the meal by opening more receptors on muscle, fat and organ cell membranes, enabling an influx of energy into cells, so that they can do work. This primary role of insulin is not a *bad* thing, but a *good* thing. We, of course, would like our cells to be able to repair themselves, produce enzymes, copy DNA, fight infection, move our bodies, think big thoughts, whatever it is they are meant to do.

Insulin's positive action, of helping energy get delivered, is not the problem.

The problem (according to the carbohydrate hypothesis) is that high insulin levels inhibit lipolysis (fat break down) and increase lipogenesis (fat creation). However, one could counter that this is not an accidental side effect of the hormone's activity, occurring only when levels rise abnormally high, but *part of its every day role* as a regulator. While sugar is available for cells to do work, there is no need to create energy from stored fat, so insulin, the hormone which responds to sugar levels, simultaneously acts also to stop fat breakdown. This coupling of actions works out very nicely. These same pathways manage energy in lean individuals as well. But the fact that one of insulin's roles in the body is to stop lipolysis and simultaneously encourage lipogenesis makes it easy to see why some would consider lowering insulin levels necessary for weight loss. We literally couldn't store fat without it.

However, there is a host of problems with this thinking, the most important of which is to realize that insulin does not act alone. Right next to the cells that produce and secrete insulin in the endocrine part of the pancreas, are cells that secrete its antidote: glucagon. Built into the system is a countermeasure that keeps insulin from performing its actions in an out of control manner. Glucagon's role is to figuratively follow insulin around and reverse each of its actions, so that they are controlled in degree and duration (think of insulin as a parent in a child's room putting all the toys away and glucagon as the toddler following her around, pulling things off the shelf almost as fast as they get stored). Additionally, Insulin itself has an indirect and delayed mechanism for ensuring it doesn't run amok. After a meal, insulin is one of the key appetite suppressing hormones in the brain. This ensures that the brain will receive a strong "stop eating" signal that is proportional to the percentage of glucose in the meal. By this negative feedback loop, insulin itself decreases future insulin secretion, through inhibiting future feeding. In addition, the baseline insulin that is secreted all day long is proportional to our body size, so insulin can be considered as a regulator of our long term weight by inhibiting appetite generally to counteract our growth. As Dan Bessesen, at the University of Colorado, mentioned to me in an interview: The quickest criticism of the low-carb diet philosophy is to ask, "Why would you want to lower one of strongest satiety signals in the body?"


## Fat Trafficking

With regard to balancing food intake with what's needed by the body, Dr. Bessesen proposes that, in addition to being able to "partition" the energy into fat cells for storage or to muscles for energy, a healthy body needs to keep track of the nutrient status of its tissues, as in, how much fat, carbohydrate and protein are needed throughout the body, at any given moment. One overlooked aspect of the scientific discussions about food intake is that the body must regulate feeding while integrating energy status signals from tissues in different nutrition states. For instance, just after a meal, the gut would be in very positive energy balance, the liver might be neutral, while the fat and muscle cells might still be energy negative because they haven't yet received the newly ingested energy. If we picture the hypothalamus in the brain as a simple "energy sensor" that tells us to eat when we are "empty" and to stop when we are "full," how would it make that decision, considering the differing nutritional states of the various tissues? Rather than just talking about hunger signals in the brain responding to a generic energy cue from the body, Dr. Bessesen proposes that it is more likely that the nutrients themselves: fat, carbohydrate and protein, are regulated.

In a 2008 article ruminating on "what's the regulated parameter" for human energy balance, Dr. Bessesen points out that fat is in much more abundant supply in the body compared to the other macronutrients. We store almost no protein. So the 50 to 60 grams we eat each day needs to be recycled about four times in 24 hours in order to achieve the build up and breakdown of complex molecules, enzymes, and tissues. There is a bit more room for flexibility with carbohydrate. We have about 800 grams (less than 2 pounds) of carbohydrate stored as glycogen in the muscles and liver, which is used for actual energy. The 200-300 grams of carbs we eat per day is about 1/4th of what's stored, so the body, naturally, would need to keep fairly tight control of carbohydrate status to prevent running too high or too low on any given day. With fat, however, a typical adult has about *150 times more* stored than is eaten daily. In terms of energy, even lean people have enough stored in the adipose for a month or two. Given these numbers, Bessesen reasons, one "might think that dietary fat would not generate much of a signal following ingestion because the change in total body lipid content produced by the fat contained in a meal is quite small." He then

61

explains why thinking that way would be false. The body actually seems just as interested in monitoring the minute-to-minute level of fat ingested, used, and moved as it is in the minute-to-minute glucose fluctuations that are so vital to our energy balance. Bessesen proposes that the ability to sense these differences (in fat availability) may be what distinguishes those prone to leanness and those prone to obesity. He contends that fat, as a nutrient used for energy, may be the most regulated factor.

Many obesity researchers talk of fat "partitioning," which is the concept that the body decides, on a constant basis, whether to deliver fat in the blood to the lean tissues for energy, or to the fat tissue for storage. The rate limiting step, in the partitioning model, is how open to absorbing fatty acids the adipose cells are compared to the muscles. If your body directs more of the energy you eat into the adipose compartment than to the lean compartment, you will become overweight or obese. But this explanation may be too simplistic, because the fat that we eat and digest and what the adipose tissue stores or releases and what the muscles use, is not permanently "partitioned" to any body compartment. In 1995, Bessesen's lab (Interview, 2013) took rats and fed them fatty rodent chow labeled with a radioactive tracer and then used fluoroscopy to see where the fat ended up. Surprisingly, after 24 hours, more than 50% of the fat was *still in the gut,* sitting in the cells that line the intestines. The researchers were able to watch as the fat made its way to the liver, then the muscle tissue, then the adipose, over many days.

A traditional view of energy balance would assume that once the fat finally reached the adipose, whether it took hours or days, that it would then be stored for use in the distant future, in a sense "locked away" until needed. But the rats showed that this isn't so. The fat was found to light up in the liver and the muscles for many days after that single meal, with the fat tissue seeming to be a net fat exporter over weeks. The initial labeled fatty acids remained detectable in the walls of the gut for as long as *one month*. This suggests that the regulation of energy is a much more complicated, nuanced, long term endeavor than a simple "go/no-go" eating decision in the brain based on hunger, or immediate energy needs.

This theoretical experiment in rats demonstrates what many scientists have argued: The adipose not a simple repository for excess energy. Furthermore, the fat itself, the stuff we eat, the free fatty acids and triglycerides that get measured in the blood, those little molecules, are much more active (and crucial to health) than we generally acknowledge. Fat circulates through the body *because we need it.* If the fatty acids were simply "excess energy," then storage would be the best thing for them. Permanent storage. But in fact, they are essential participants in our complex metabolism, helping to regulate the energy needed for all the reactions which occur in our organs. So the person who experiences an ongoing growth of his adipose tissue is not dealing strictly with an excess calorie problem. Nor is it a problem of simple partitioning, because the partitioning is only temporary. The fat we eat goes into the gut, gets absorbed and stored by the cells lining the intestines, enters the blood, the liver, the muscle, the adipose, then keeps circulating between those cell types. The fat comes and goes through the adipose cells, just like it does the liver (and probably muscle). It is the coming and going of the fat, how it is trafficked, which decides how lean or fatty our body will become.

## Is Lowering Insulin Necessary for Weight Loss?

In September of 2015, Kevin Hall and colleagues published an article in *Cell Metabolism* entitled, "Calorie for Calorie, Dietary Fat Restriction Results in More Body Fat Loss than Carbohydrate Restriction in People with Obesity." This was not a diet intervention study, but a mechanistic test of whether altering macronutrients might differentially affect metabolism. The researchers took 19 volunteers and studied them in the highly controlled circumstances of a "metabolic ward" which has the ability to assess total energy expenditure for an individual's body. Each participant did both diets, which were 30% reductions of total calories either through carb reduction or fat reduction. A host of variables was assessed before and after the six day diet periods, including body fat, insulin, glucose, as well as several of the hormones that mediate hunger in the gut (such as Ghrelin and GIP), but most importantly, they computed the oxidation of nutrients.

This is something that can't be done in the usual diet study which pits one diet concept against another and decides success based on participants' weight at six months. This study was run in these highly controlled conditions in order to test some specific contentions of the carbohydrate hypothesis:

*—Does low-carb dieting alter nutrient oxidation?*

*—Does that response lead to greater fat loss?*

*—Can weight loss occur in circumstances of normal insulin levels?*

What the authors concluded, is that you *can* lose weight on a low-fat diet which does *not* act through changing insulin. In fact, they found, by looking specifically at fat oxidation, that more fat is burned by restricting fat intake than restricting carbohydrate intake. While on low-fat diets, the volunteers had a net fat loss of 89 grams per day and only 53 g/day on low-carb. These rates of fat oxidation were calculated by a combination of validated methods using indirect calorimetry (oxygen in . . . $CO_2$ out) combined with measures of 24 hour nitrogen losses in urine.

During the low-fat phase, participants had no change from baseline in the metabolism of any macronutrient: rate of fat oxidation, carbohydrate oxidation and protein oxidation did not significantly adapt to cutting 800 calories per day. As a result, during the low-fat weeks, the subjects lost very close to the theoretical maximum of 800 calories worth of fat per day (765 +/-37).

During the low-carb phase, on the other hand, there were significant metabolic adaptations. Subjects were found to have ramped up fat oxidation by 403 cal/day and decreased carbohydrate oxidation by 520 grams per day. This would seem like validation of the low-carb hypothesis, right? Everybody switched to "fat burning mode" when the carbs were cut. But the switch wasn't efficient. The slowing of carbohydrate burning *overbalanced* the increase in fat burning, such that *overall rate of oxidation* of nutrients was slower while

65

on a lower-carb diet than baseline. They still lost fat, but not as much as theoretically possible from cutting 800 calories, because of this inefficiency.

The low-carb diet produced less fat loss than the low-fat diet. But that is probably not the most important point in the paper, since the difference was pretty small. Because this was a study of *how* we lose weight, specifically looking at low-carb diet recommendations, a much more interesting point is that insulin was entirely unchanged in the low-fat group.

I asked Kevin Hall whether this meant that he'd disproved the carbohydrate hypothesis:

*"The reduced-carb diet does everything that the proponents of low-carb diets claim: it reduces insulin secretion, it increases fat oxidation AND it leads to fat loss. But this study was designed to look at another diet in comparison: If you don't decrease insulin because you don't decrease carbs, can you also get fat loss?*

*"Some folks have made the very strong claim that if you don't reduce insulin by reducing carbs, in particular refined carbs, then you can't lose fat from the body. And this study clearly demonstrates that that is not true. Insulin secretion went down in the low-carb group by 22% and stayed the same in the low-fat group."*

As the low-carb researchers close in on "proving" their hypothesis, this study gives an important pause and demands that we remember the big picture. Showing that insulin is the proximate necessary hormone enabling fat storage is not the same as showing that it *causes* fat storage. The focus on insulin's action as the key step in weight gain ignores that there is a vast host of signals regulating hunger, digestion, and energy usage: ghrelin tells the brain that the stomach is empty; insulin can't stop it. CCK and PYY are secreted by the small intestine. They act to slow stomach emptying and tell the brain that nutrient levels are rising. Insulin doesn't affect them. Leptin and adiponectin are secreted by fat cells to give feedback on whether we are growing heavier over time. Insulin doesn't change what they do. Cortisol from the adrenal glands promotes a stress response that causes many people to eat more. It does this without asking insulin's permission. Thyroid hormone turns up the metabolic action of almost all of our cells and fluctuations in its level can cause dramatic weight loss or weight gain . . . again without any input from insulin. None of these hormones are related to the carbohydrate level in the diet, either. They are simply acting outside of the focus of the carbohydrate hypothesis.

**Why Intelligent People Disagree**

The apparent disagreement between those who point out insulin's key role in fat storage and those who believe it's more complicated than that, is not, in my opinion, a disagreement about scientific facts. The two camps are really talking about different things. The low-carb advocates are focused on the major hormonal steps of regulation, while the critics are generally more interested in appetite control and whole body energy status. In simple terms, the debate is frequently framed: "Is a calorie a calorie?" But really no debate is possible when one group is looking at cellular signaling in the liver and the other is looking at hunger regulation in the brain. Some bridging of the two areas of interest is needed to get a complete view of the obesity problem. From this standpoint, I think it's more appropriate to consider insulin necessary, but not sufficient, to cause obesity. It can also be said that glucose is necessary, but not sufficient and dietary fat is necessary, but not sufficient. All three must be present. But for insulin to do its job of promoting fat storage, the appetite must allow the excess energy to enter in the first place. We are still at a loss to explain (using low-carb thinking) why our intake has increased and why many individuals feel very unsatisfied on a low-carbohydrate diet.

The carbohydrate hypothesis has the biochemistry nailed down. I don't believe there is much debate on that. It is in proposing dietary solutions to alter this biochemistry that low-carb diet advocates run afoul of the scientists holding a more traditional view. Acknowledging that glucose is the primary stimulator of insulin does not mean that we have to eliminate, or even drastically reduce, carbohydrate in the diet. By all measures, the increase in carbohydrate, which is associated with the increase in obesity rates, is a subtle change that has crept into our diet at a very slow rate. We've increased carbohydrates perhaps 5-10%, or about 50 grams per day, gradually, over four decades. Why would we need to all but eliminate a nutrient that accounts for nearly half of our energy requirement?

By focusing too narrowly on just part of the picture, the carbohydrate hypothesis fails to account for all of the other pathways that affect our weight, most importantly, neglecting to account for appetite mechanisms that act to balance out unbalanced diet approaches, including

Atkins. This leads to frustration in many individuals following a low-carb diet, who state, "Sure it works, but I'm starving!" In my experience, patients typically consider low-carb living a temporary approach to achieve quick weight loss, rather than a sustainable way of eating to maintain health. I believe that the discussion of the counter-measures above helps to explain why. While it may be scientifically valid to propose that we reduce carbs to reduce insulin to reduce fat stores . . . Immediately, the counter-regulatory measures, working via nutrient sensing, variations in metabolism and appetite control, will induce us, through hunger (and specific cravings) to rebalance our feeding until our weight is restored. When this happens, the person dieting blames himself for giving in to sugar cravings. Perhaps he should blame the diet which seems designed to provoke sugar cravings.

The arguments above don't disprove the carbohydrate hypothesis; they merely cast doubt on the completeness of the explanation, particularly the proposed solution to the problem, which is to eliminate a very long list of foods. Gary Taubes wrote a second book on the carbohydrate hypothesis titled simply *Why We Get Fat*. This was a pared-down version of the larger thesis of *Good Calories, Bad Calories*, intended to be a more readable text for a broader audience. He jokes that it was written in response to doctors who wanted an easier version to give to patients . . . and for patients who wanted an easier version to give to their doctors. However, the question posed in the title is not answered in the book. The carbohydrate explanation of obesity, regardless of the level of detail and clarity of explanation, is a description of "how" we become obese, not "why." It explains the mechanisms and the processes that control energy and how they function on a fundamental level. But it does not account for the reason that these processes have gone awry, aside from proposing that carbohydrates act as an unbalancing influence. We are still left to wonder why humans over-ingest carbohydrates in the first place. It is not typical for an animal to behave for long periods of time in a manner that makes it sicker. We are adapted to eat in certain ways and even in the context of an obesity pandemic, our regulation is almost intact, remaining within 10 or 20 calories of what we should be eating daily. Why are we suddenly unable to adjust to the food that is available to us?

Contrary to what Dr. Atkins claimed about his "vast majority" of clients, many people feel terribly hungry and dissatisfied without simple sugars and complex carbohydrates. People don't crave these foods because they are stupid, or weak-willed. The food companies haven't been making them because they have evil intentions. We started milling grain 5000 years ago and our weight only began to rise 40 years ago. Carbohydrates are a staple of the human diet because we operate quite well on them. We don't need to *eliminate* them; we need to *balance* them with our other nutrients. To continue our current obesity discussion, we need to look elsewhere to uncover the reason for our increase in weight. Carbohydrate consumption has risen over the last 40 years and supplied each of us with at least 200 calories more energy per day. The relationship between the carbs, the calories, and our weight is clear. The question is not "how" we became obese, but "why?"

# References:

Atkins, Robert C. *Dr. Atkins' New Diet Revolution.* Maryland: M. Evans Publishing; 2002.

Taubes, Gary. *Good Calories, Bad Calories.* New York: Random House; 2007.

Ebbeling, CB, et. al. Effects of dietary composition on energy expenditure during weight-loss maintenance. *JAMA* 2012, 307(24): 2627-34.

Foster, GD, et. al. A randomized trial of a low-carbohydrate diet for obesity. *NEJM* 2003, 348(21): 2082-2090.

Yang, MU and Van Itallie, TB. Composition of weight lost during short-term weight reduction. *Journal of Clinical Investigation* 1976, 58(3): 722-730.

Austin GL, Ogden LG and Hill JO. Trends in carbohydrate, fat and protein intakes and association with energy intake in normal-weight, overweight and obese individuals: 1971-2006. *American Journal of Clinical Nutrition* 2011, 93(4): 836-43.

Westman EC, et. al. Low-carbohydrate nutrition and metabolism. *American Journal of Clinical Nutrition* 2007, 86(2): 276-84.

Bessesen D., Regulation of body weight: what is the regulated parameter? *Physiology and Behavior* 2011, 104(4): 599-607.

Bessesen EH, et. al. Trafficking of dietary fat in lean rats. Obesity Reviews 1995, 3(2):191-203.

Hall, KD, et. al. Calorie for calorie, dietary fat restriction results in more body fat loss than carbohydrate restriction in people with obesity. *Cell Metabolism.* Published online August 13, 2015.

Taubes, Gary. *Why We Get Fat.* New York: Random House; 2011.

# Chapter 4

## The Protein Leverage Hypothesis

Kevin Hall and Carson Chow demonstrated (in a 2010 paper) that the rise of obesity prevalence in the U.S. since the 1970s can be attributed to an increase in consumption of just seven calories per day, per person. This is calculated by taking the average increase of energy stored in the heavier adult bodies of the present day, divided by the very long time frame it took for the change to occur.

The seven calories, on a daily basis, refers to the excess one would eat *at that weight*. Once we grow bigger, of course, the bigger body requires more calories to support it, so one would need a slow increase in food quantity over time to remain seven calories in excess daily. When we look at the change in overall daily calorie consumption over the last 40 years (and this is the number we would need to target if we want to change obesity in the population), we now eat an average of 220 calories extra, per day, to maintain our bigger size (rounding off NHANES data). So the change we are hoping to produce in the individual, depending upon where they are in their weight gain journey, would be somewhere between seven and 220 calories per day.

This is somewhere between a sip and an entire 20-ounce bottle of Coca-Cola. There is a general misperception that very heavy people must eat much more than slimmer people, but these numbers demonstrate just how subtle the difference can be. The calorie problem, and any proposed solution, are both too small to accurately assess on a day-to-day basis. Our ability to control our weight is limited by this fact.

To make progress, we must hope that there is something that we can do regarding *what* we are eating, that might control *how much*. Low-carbohydrate diets seem moderately more effective than low-fat diets, but neither approach solves the obesity problem, because they both produce very small amounts of weight loss and fail when participants go back to "eating as usual." If low-carbohydrate diets show all the metabolic advantages we reviewed last chapter and work better than low-fat or low-calorie diets, why are they not a definitive, permanent solution for a greater number of people? Why do they produce average weight losses that would still qualify as "not even disappointing"?

## We Are Asking the Wrong Questions

One reason that we don't find *any* single diet strategy that works for everyone is that these strategies are targeted at individuals deliberately making conscious changes in their behavior. They depend upon each person learning and implementing solutions to their own particular weight problem, as if there was something peculiarly wrong with their unique metabolism. But the shifts that have occurred regarding our nutrient intake suggest that it is changes at the level of the entire food supply that should attract our attention for obesity causation and treatment.

In 2005, David Raubenheimer and Stephen Simpson quietly proposed a novel solution to the mystery of the obesity epidemic and coined the term "protein leverage" to re-frame the question of human obesity in terms reflecting animals interacting with their ecology to get the nutrition they need. I say "quietly" because, despite actively searching the obesity literature and attending a wide array of conferences on nutrition science, I'd never heard the term until seven years after their first paper on protein leverage came out. In a series of observations, experiments and sometimes abstruse articles, Raubenheimer, Simpson and colleagues have shown that many species, including humans, regulate food intake by how much protein is needed to maximize health and reproduction. The idea of "leverage" is used to explain the fact that small changes in protein availability can trigger large changes in animal behavior. When protein becomes less available, fruit flies will hold off on mating, humans will overeat and crickets will become cannibals.

I first became aware of their ideas in March of 2012, while trying to find academic articles studying "higher protein" diets as opposed to "low-carb," "Paleo," "Zone," or "Atkins" diets. I was looking for scientific validation of the diet scheme that I'd been advocating, which was to hold calories a bit lower than the patient's usual eating, while increasing the proportion of protein consumed. I had come to this philosophy not by reading about it, but by reviewing the diet records of my patients. These almost uniformly showed that people with weight problems under-ingest protein compared to even the conservative USDA recommendations.

When we tried to decrease calories through simple portion control, the problem of low-protein got worse, since smaller portions of low-protein foods just reduced all nutrients indiscriminately. This, again, was made clear by looking at the breakdown of nutrients in the patient food logs. To combat this, I began to recommend increasing the protein percentage. As I did that, I started seeing more positive results with my patients. I noted that the beneficial effect of the higher protein approach seemed to correlate with many popular approaches found in diet books. However, I'd never been able to swallow the strange Atkins assumption that carbohydrates are a "bad" food, or that we should all eat like cave men. Few naturally skinny humans need to purposely restrict carbohydrate to remain lean, I reasoned, and nearly every animal eats some combination of fat, carbohydrate and protein and naturally approaches optimum health without excluding tasty food. Something always seemed missing until I stumbled onto Simpson's and Raubenheimer's papers.

Unfortunately for the average U.S. layperson, these scientists work in ecology and zoology in Australia. So, while their ideas have appeared in recognized journals related to humans, such as *Obesity Reviews,* their theory has not caused much of a stir here. Because they are trying to bring together insights regarding many different species, the implications of their work are a bit buried in their papers in terminology and a graphical model they've invented called the "geometric framework."

In 2012, the two scientists finally put together the major findings regarding protein leverage into a beautiful, readable book titled *The Nature of Nutrition-a unifying framework from animal adaptation to human obesity*. While the geometric framework is still the centerpiece of their theory, the depth and breadth of the book bring even non-visual and non-mathematical readers to the understanding that protein may be the key to understanding the cause of our weight problems.

They demonstrate that most animals balance carbohydrate, fat and protein ratios within a fairly narrow space of optimal function. The animals either find themselves in an environment in which the natural balance of nutrients leads to good health without any regulation, or they regulate by choosing amongst a variety of imbalanced foods in order to get to the ideal. Through observation of how species act in the wild and by purposely changing the diet of study animals, the authors find, again and again, that species have an ability to detect what's needed for optimum health and to generally feed in a way that maximizes fitness. When this can't be done, the individuals of a given species tend to adapt in a uniform manner, for example: sacrificing some reproductive health for living longer, or losing some size advantage to maintain energy. They call the observed adaptation the "Rule of Compromise" for that species.

Another possible means for overcoming poor nutrition in the local environment is to just pick up and move. When the environment is altered (as when seasonal changes cause protein to fall, or the food supply runs out) many insects and animals migrate. The most graphic example is the story of Mormon crickets, which form large migration clusters when protein runs low. The authors were able to show that the starving insects were driven to search not just for food, but *high protein* food, to the point that they would pass up many possible sources of energy (for instance, the grasses in the migration path) to get to an improved nutritional environment. So starved for protein were these insects, that if one of their brethren dropped dead from exhaustion and starvation, they preferred the fallen as a food source to the high-carbohydrate fare along the way.

The authors work their way up the food chain through salmon, rats and monkeys to finally explain what's going on with humans. We, like many other species, seem particularly regulated by the amount of protein in the diet. While self-regulating human populations across the world and across several decades can be shown to eat a wide range of fat and carbohydrate calories, the amount of protein in the diet is nearly always 15% of the total. The authors compared the composition of the diets found in several countries to show that humans tolerate very wide ranges of carbohydrate and fat in the diet while remaining in good health. Together, fat and carbohydrate consistently add up to 85% of calories, but there is little pattern as to how much each supplies of that 85%. Populations that live near the sea tend to fill much of the 85% with fat calories, while landlocked peoples balance it out with carbohydrate from grains or tubers. This suggests that carbohydrate and fat are interchangeable sources of "energy" while protein is the prime necessary nutrient the body will not go without. In balanced, naturally regulated human populations with stable weights, the 15% protein number is found again and again.

So, what does the science of nutritional ecology have to say about the "obesity epidemic" in industrialized countries? Simpson and Raubenheimer show that we are acting just like the crickets (well, not *just* like the crickets, thank goodness) and we are defending our protein target by a natural adjustment to a changed environment. USDA figures and other databases (FAOSTAT) show that the relative proportion of available protein in the food supply has decreased from 14-15% (just what we need) to 12.5%. This leaves us to feed in a sub-optimal environment in which the amount of protein we need to maintain health is harder to obtain. In fact, if we don't consciously seek out protein and instead eat freely from the available food supply, we are in essence *forced* to over-consume fat and carbohydrate calories to reach our protein goal.

Because protein has been diluted by carbohydrate in the modern food supply, we must eat more carbohydrate to gain limited protein. Because food is so easy to obtain for most of us, we've made the switch to these lower protein foods at the expense of a couple hundred extra calories a day without noticing much has changed . . . except of course, our weight, which we've sort of been puzzled about, but not too puzzled to stop seeking the nutrients we need.

## How Does Protein Control Food Intake?

The insight of these scientists is in the concept of "protein leverage." Historically, most researchers have discounted the importance of protein's contribution to the obesity problem because it is such a small percentage of our total intake and because it is so constant across time and geography. Those two facts have made it very difficult to see that protein is actually the root cause of the obesity problem. *Because* we have to keep protein constant and *because* it is such a small component of overall intake, small changes in the percentage of protein have mathematical leverage to affect calorie consumption beyond expectations. In order to make up for a 1.5% decrease in the protein content in the diet, a medium sized person must consume *14% more total calories* to reach the nutritional target.

Those calories currently come from an increase in carbohydrate, making it seem as if the carbohydrate itself has caused our obesity problem. But the protein leverage framework argues that the calories could just as easily come from fat, or a combination of both. Their role in this narrative is only as "non-protein energy." Protein amount is small, but it can leverage large changes in the diet. The following example demonstrates the type of math found in their book:

A 150 pound man is at a stable weight eating 2400 calories per day with 14% of energy (336 cals) coming from protein. The other 86% of energy (2064 cals) is made up of fat and carbohydrate.

The 336 calories of protein represent 84 grams needed daily, his protein target. If the amount of protein available decreases from 14% to 12.5%, he will have to make due with 75 grams per day. Or . . . he could begin to overeat the protein-dilute food to maintain the protein that his muscles and organs require for optimum function. How many calories does he need to eat daily to maintain his 84 grams of protein?

84g = 336 protein calories. 336 is 14% of 2400.

If protein is reduced to 12.5%, what number is 336 12.5% of?

336 cals divided by 12.5% = 2,688 cals.

So if protein need is absolute and our bodies will technically be starving without our daily quantity, the internal regulation of appetite will unconsciously drive this man's consumption from 2400 to 2688 per day to stay healthy. Perhaps not coincidentally, the number of calories in this example correlates fairly well to the amount of reported calorie increase in the American diet over the last 30 years.

Why would the body do this? Choose to be obese, or even diabetic, due to a change in the food environment? Because obesity is quite sustainable and doesn't really decrease reproduction or fitness in a way that matters as much as protein starvation would. Diabetes, certainly, can be a difficult state to be in, but it's preferable to letting the body remain low on protein, which would lead to poor functioning of muscles and organs, as well as reduced reproduction and longevity. Given the available options in the current food environment, the strategy we have adopted is to consume excess calories in order to gain the scarcer protein . . . and suffer the consequences.

Simpson and Raubenheimer call this the "Rule of Compromise" for human nutrition. We are obese because it is a reasonable trade off, given our choices. Keep in mind: These are not conscious choices, but internal regulatory drives much too subtle, persistent and powerful to be over-ruled by our determination. You can diet for five or six months, but this system keeps track of what's best for you over an entire lifetime. It keeps track of what's best for our species as a whole, perhaps over evolutionary timescales.

Other theories of obesity attribute our over-consumption of calories to conscious or unconscious preference for sugar or fat. We are thought to be programmed by evolutionary pressure to take in calories when they are available, because famine is thought to have been common in our ancestors. By this thinking, some individuals and more notably, some populations, have "thrifty genes" that make them want calories whenever they are available. The protein leverage hypothesis does not disprove the thrifty gene theory; it complements it. But protein leverage thinking proposes that it is not simply more calories we seek, but more protein calories. If protein is the ultimate target for consumption, trumping our other needs, then carbohydrates or fat are being over-consumed presently not because they were once rare and our internal regulation treasures them, but because they are in the way of the protein we need. This enables us to propose solutions for obesity that do not require speculating on the dietary habits of hunter-gatherers.

Protein leverage, through a dispassionate comparison of humans with other animals, encourages us to think of obesity as an adaptation to the environment, rather than a disease state. In order to stay healthy, we must meet our protein target. To reach the target with our current food supply, we must overeat. To handle the excess calories, we store some as fat. Our ability to store fat is almost unlimited, so we grow indefinitely larger. With regard to handling energy, however, our adaptation is not unlimited. With regard to increased fat and carbohydrate intake, for a time the body responds with a higher insulin level, which pushes blood sugar into muscles and other tissues. But, as this plays out over many years, our bodies become less sensitive to insulin's action.

Insulin's regulatory mechanisms are considered by some to be "overused" by constant presence of glucose in the diet, making it less and less effective. Specifically, muscle and organ cells become unable to respond to the signal to open glucose channels to transport sugar through the membrane. When we reach that stage, we are stuck with the carbohydrate, in the form of glucose, remaining in the blood or spilled in the urine as waste. We have become diabetic. Obesity and diabetes are simply the result of necessary over-consumption by the body seeking adequate nutrition. Perhaps neither problem would occur if we supplied enough necessary protein to the body in the first place.

This conclusion, that our need for protein is controlling our feeding, while counter-intuitive at first, makes a number of other questions easier to answer:

—Why are we all eating so much? *Because we're starving (for protein).*

—Why can't we lose weight by eating less? *Because that makes the starvation worse.*

—Why do we regain lost weight? *The body is counteracting the starvation.*

—Why does weight gain seem to accelerate as one grows larger? *Because the heavier body needs even more protein, so must increase consumption faster.*

When we put protein at the center of our focus, the futility of simply eating less, particularly "portion control," becomes obvious: the body is actually more balanced, nutritionally, at the heavier weight, since it got to that weight by prioritizing protein. If you reduce how much you're eating, including protein, the body is wise to resist. It doesn't care as much about the number of pounds up or down as it does about the protein. Every time we reduce calories using a "balanced" approach, we reduce the number of protein grams even further and our body, naturally, compensates . . . just like an insect, fish or primate living in the wild.

To accept this proposed explanation of human obesity requires us to recognize that we share some of our primitive drives and the mechanisms for survival with the rest of the animal kingdom. The most humbling comparison is to consider the slime mold. This particular organism is literally a "blob" without organs, brain, nervous system, or even separate cells. Through very careful observation and experimentation with different nutrients, Dussutour and colleagues, in 2010, were able to show that slime molds slowly move toward particular nutrient targets over time. The "blob" was shown to have particular nutrition needs that it was able to satisfy by growing toward its preferred food over several days. Rather than being humbled by our similarity to slime molds, I simply think: "If blobs can do it, certainly we humans must be capable of it too."

In determining the winner of the debate regarding obesity causation and the best diet for weight loss, I believe that Simpson and Raubenheimer's work allows us to finally settle the question in such a way that everyone can be happy: The low-carb advocates are correct. The low-fat advocates are correct. The low-calorie advocates are correct. Even the high protein weight lifter types are correct. They are each correct due to the underlying principle of protein leverage.

You can either decrease fat, decrease carbs, or even decrease both together in a low-calorie approach, as long as you keep protein constant. Protecting the lean tissues of the body enables weight loss to proceed more easily. When low-fat diets work, when low-carb diets work, when low-calorie diets work, it is because they maintain or raise the protein quantity in the diet. Simpson and Raubenheimer consider those diets to be special cases of the general rule of protein leverage.

This simple proposal, that protein in the diet regulates how much we need to eat, is different from the other proposals about obesity. The high-fat hypothesis, the carbohydrate hypothesis and the "calorie is a calorie" hypothesis, all deal with obesity as a disease. They seek the explanation for a particular problem that is occurring to a particular group of humans at this one time in our history. The protein leverage hypothesis is not just an explanation of obesity. It proposes to explain how our nutrition, in general, is regulated and how it relates to nutrition patterns observed in other species.

The authors are not simply proposing a new way of looking at obesity, they are asserting that they've discovered a "rule" of nutrition (although they are careful to couch their proposal as a "framework"). If the

85

proposal holds up to analysis over time, it would be, by my reasoning, really only the second rule of nutrition to be discovered. The first would be that energy into the organism must equal energy out (with allowances for losses through heat and waste). Moreover, if it is truly a rule, we should expect to see it manifesting wherever we look at diet.

## Looking for Protein Leverage in the Medical Literature

In the paper by Austin and colleagues that we discussed in the previous chapter, regarding NHANES data, the authors noted that protein and fat, measured by grams, remained constant while carbohydrate was the only macronutrient that quantitatively increased from 1970's to present. They didn't speculate on the cause of the change and don't make reference to the idea of protein leverage. However, included in their discussion of various analytic models they ran on the dataset, there is a mention of a relationship very much in support of the Simpson/Raubenheimer thesis:

*"One of the most striking findings of this study was the consistently strong and negative association with increasing percentage calories from protein and daily energy intake across all 3 BMI categories . . . if protein was increased from 15% to 25% of energy intake in an obese individual, this would be expected to be associated with a decrease in energy intake of 438 calories (if substituted for carbohydrates) or 620 calories (if substituted for fat)."* —Austin 2009

Austin includes references to other studies which deal with high vs. low-protein diets, but again, seems to have no knowledge of Simpson and Raubenheimer's work at the time of writing. *The Nature of Nutrition* was not published until a year later, so we can speculate that Austin stumbled into this example of the rule of compromise, by scrutinizing the data and applying careful reason.

In 2015, a review of the effect of higher protein diets, published in the *International Journal of Obesity* by Arne Astrup, found evidence for protein advantage in adults who had lost weight and subsequently on their children. This European, multi-site study was designed to test diets of different protein quantity and carbohydrate quality on weight loss and normal daily intake of calories in families. An increase of 5% protein in the diet resulted in significantly less energy intake and spontaneous weight loss in overweight and obese children who were not formally following a weight loss diet. Dr. Astrup noted:

*"The most significant outcome of the DioGenes study was that very subtle changes in diet composition with respect to protein and carbohydrates seem to have a major impact on spontaneous caloric intake." —Astrup 2015*

Again, there is no mention of protein leverage per se and no references to Simpson, Raubenheimer, or their colleagues in the quoted references.

James Hill and his colleagues who follow the successful individuals in the National Weight Control Registry published an analysis in the journal *Obesity* in

2012, in which they sought to characterize diet styles so that we may begin to customize diet advice more appropriately to certain types and dispositions. Previous papers from the national weight control registry could be used to argue that macronutrients *don't matter* for weight loss: The members of the registry don't subscribe to any unified diet philosophy. Half of them use commercial weight loss programs, half don't. Most exercise, but many don't. Some have dieted many times, some were successful on the first attempt. It's hard to look at these researchers' papers and conclude that there is a particular method that is common to all successful weight loss participants.

However, in their 2012 paper, the authors included a table with the macronutrient breakdown of the groups they sought to characterize. While the four subgroups differed in the percentage of calories that come from carbohydrates (48-54%) and fat (26-31%), they all fell into a very narrow range for protein percent: 18, 18, 19, and 19%. This isn't remarked upon in the discussion; it's simply listed like everything else, but it is relevant to our current discussion. Across human populations, both in terms of geography and time, we find that protein is nearly always 14-15% of calories. Here we find a group of extremely successful weight loss registry members who consistently report eating 4-5% more protein than the average typical human diet. While this finding is outside of the interest of the authors of the paper, it provides some useful numbers for testing our thesis.

Protein leverage would predict that if you shift a person from 14-15% of a 2600 calorie diet (averages from NHANES) up to 19%, then, in order keep grams of protein constant, the body would need to decrease calorie consumption by 410 cal/day, just to avoid protein excess. This alone might be the permanent compensation that has made 50-100 pound weight loss possible for these individuals. What makes this more interesting is that the participants were not specifically encouraged to eat more protein. These are the self-directed individuals who have signed up for Dr. Hill's registry, who have been noted to use all manner of methods. Yet, they all eat the same in terms of protein, while allowing the non-protein energy of carbs and fat to fluctuate. Could protein leverage be silently driving the success of these individuals while they believe they are purposely reducing calories, avoiding fat, "doing paleo" or any number of other methods?

Alison Gosby and colleagues published a systematic review in 2014 which sought to quantify the protein leverage effect found within already published weight loss trials. After sifting through 2000 studies, and applying rigid criteria, they found 38 which adequately compared and reported on diets of varying protein composition and daily intakes. When they plotted calories against protein, they found, as expected, a negative correlation between protein and calories. As protein rose from 10 to 20%, the effect of protein leverage was fairly profound: calories decreased approximately 40% on average across the study groups (my interpretation, based on dataset). Above 20 percent, increasing protein further had significantly less impact, implying perhaps, a threshold effect, beyond which the relationship becomes less important.

**Looking for Protein Leverage in Diet Journals**

When you are in medical practice, you don't have access to the type of information on your patients that researchers have on their subjects. While I had intuitively stumbled on the protein leverage effect early on and found that increasing protein seemed to help patients, I had not actually measured its influence on day-to-day calories. Once I became aware of the research discussed above, I decided to test the protein leverage hypothesis more formally with one of my very successful weight loss patients, whom we will call Andy. Andy came to the clinic weighing 480 pounds. He had never successfully dieted. I don't remember what brought him in at first. There was no particular new health crisis like a heart attack or diagnosis of diabetes. He was married, an engineer, and healthy, aside from his weight. At any rate, Andy really seemed to understand what I explained about protein leverage. Being an engineer, he also happened to love my suggestion to rigorously track calories, carbs, fats and protein amounts using one of the commercially available internet tools. This was something I recommended to all patients, but enthusiasms differ and certainly no one ever provided me a dataset quite like Andy's. His weight came off fast and as he got excited, he got more interested in the mechanisms. As he got more interested, he got better at controlling what he ate and how closely he measured. Not content with the graphs available with the internet site and its phone app, he began transferring all the calorie and nutrient data into excel, so we could do our own analyses. We were able to test the accuracy of his tracking by using the NIDDK weight simulator tool to predict his weight loss at each monthly visit. Andy treated his obesity as a math problem, just like the NIH researchers and the protein leverage scientists. It worked tremendously well and he reached a normal weight (for his height) in about two and a half years.

One of the things Andy and I did was to assess how well his dataset corroborated the protein leverage hypothesis. I asked him, in his graphing efforts, if he would send me a chart of protein percentage plotted against calories consumed on a daily basis. Although he was a star patient, even *he* had variability in what he ate day-to-day. I assumed that high protein days would be lower calorie than low-protein days. Protein leverage proposes that they are inversely related and protein leverage sure seemed to be working for him. If ever we could get an honest assessment of this principle working on an individual level, I figured Andy would be the ideal candidate. He recalibrated all the data points he had collected up to that date to compare protein percentage to calories. He brought back the following at his next visit:

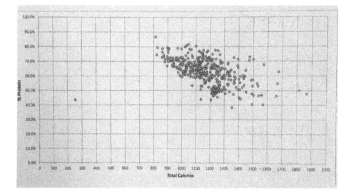

This showed exactly what protein leverage would predict: the higher the protein percentage on any given day, the fewer calories Andy consumed. Clearly, in this journal, high protein meant low-calories. I sent the graph to a colleague who replied, "Wow . . . looks too good to be true."

I gave this some thought. Andy knew what we were trying to do. It was quite possible that he was simply having "good" days and "bad" days. On a good day, he followed directions by eating more protein *and* keeping calories down, through conscious effort. On a bad day, he ate less protein and indulged a little more. Since he was in on the theory, I couldn't completely trust that his results represented a hidden rule of nutrition. So next I spoke with a developer of a new diet tracking app which was in beta-testing at the time. I had been informally advising him while he convinced friends, family, and co-workers to begin testing the app and website. I asked him to find five people for whom he had 90 days in a row of consistent tracking and send me the raw numbers. Setting up the same correlation plots that we did with Andy, we found:

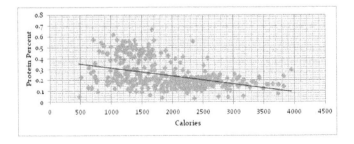

*Protein is inversely proportional to calories (correlation: -0.307)*

While the trend is not a dramatic as Andy's, it clearly suggests that with a very high protein percentage, such as over 40% it is very hard to overeat. Low-protein days seem to allow a wide variety of possible calorie ingestion.

Next we looked at the correspondence between carbohydrate and calories. We found:

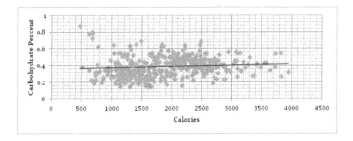

*Carbohydrate intake shows no observable effect on calories (correlation: 0.009)*

Finally, we assessed the correlation between fat and calorie consumption:

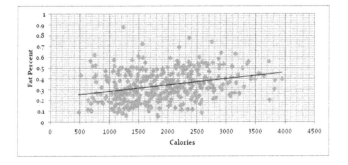

*Fat shows a positive effect on calories (correlation: 0.273)*

These graphs suggest, for this group, that protein varies with fat as the non-protein energy source, rather than carbohydrate. These data are just a small random sample and can't really test any hypothesis. I include them as an example of how macronutrients affect free living individuals. If protein leverage works as proposed, it should be detectable in this type of observational dataset. One reason this suggests to me that we are on to something important is that we do not know the motivation of the individuals who were creating the data. They were simply testers of a new product. We don't even know whether their goal was weight loss, weight maintenance, or just to mess around with a new toy. It seems unlikely that any of them were purposely testing the protein leverage hypothesis. Yet here they were, following its rule.

The proponents of a low-carbohydrate diet for obesity believe that switching from a belief system that blames dietary fat for obesity to one that blames carbohydrate for obesity would represent a major change in our thinking —a "paradigm shift." In a way, this is perhaps true, if we take it to mean that we will now focus on how fat cells are regulated, rather than simply trying to calculate or control "calories in/calories out." But to me, fat vs. carbs is not a terribly exciting debate. Researchers will soon run some more careful equal-calorie studies and pick the winner. A real change in thinking, worthy of the overused term "paradigm shift" in obesity research, would be to transition from behavioral, psychological and internal biological explanations to consider obesity a problem of ecology, as Simpson and Raubenheimer suggest. Perhaps with this wider scope, we may truly see where our nutrition has gone wrong.

## References:

Simpson, SJ and Raubenheimer, D. Obesity: The protein leverage hypothesis. *Obesity Reviews* 2005, 6: 133-144.

Simpson, Steven and Raubenheimer, David. *The Nature of Nutrition: A Unifying Framework from Animal Adaptation to Human Obesity.* Princeton University Press, 2012.

Dussutour, A. et. al. Amoeboid organism solves complex nutritional challenges. *PNAS* 2010, 107(10): 4607-4611.

Ogden LG, et al. Cluster analysis of the National Weight Control Registry to identify distinct subgroups successful at maintaining weight loss. *Obesity* 2012, 20(10): 2039-47.

Austin GL, Ogden LG and Hill JO. Trends in carbohydrate, fat and protein intakes and association with energy intake in normal-weight, overweight and obese individuals: 1971-2006. *American Journal of Clinical Nutrition* 2011, 93(4): 836-43.

Astrup, A. et. al. The role of higher protein diets in weight control and obesity related co-morbidities. *International Journal of Obesity* 2015, 39(5): 721-726.

Gosby, AK, et. al. Protein leverage and energy intake. *Obesity Reviews* 2014, 15: 183-191.

# Chapter 5

## Is Diabetes a Surgical Condition?

A new patient sits across from me in the exam room, confused and frustrated at her lack of progress trying to lose weight for the last 30 years. 200 pounds too heavy, diagnosed with type 2 diabetes, high cholesterol, hypertension, sleep apnea, infertility, and osteoarthritis. She needs knee replacements, but is too heavy to be approved for the surgery. She asks me, the "weight loss doctor," what my plan is for her. And I think: "What does it take to get referred to a bariatric surgeon in this town?"

I've been interested in obesity since I began medical practice 15 years ago, but I have to admit that I believed it to be a lifestyle and behavioral disorder until about 7 years ago, when I learned about bariatric surgery at an American Diabetes Association meeting. I was lucky enough to be in a session hosted by some of the pioneering surgeons and researchers in the field. They described their initial reaction to the first patient with type 2 diabetes who underwent gastric bypass surgery.

They had presumed that as the patient lost weight, his metabolism would improve and that they would eventually be able to reduce or even eliminate the patient's insulin. What happened instead was that the patient's blood sugar normalized and insulin became unnecessary while he was *still in the hospital.* In a matter of days, the "insulin resistance" that we consider causative for type 2 diabetes, as if by magic, resolved. The patient's natural ability to sense incoming nutrients, secrete insulin to manage those nutrients, and the body's ability to accept the action of insulin, all normalized within the course of a week. The surgeons were, to say the least, a bit surprised.

Surprised and excited. So they performed bariatric surgery on a second type 2 diabetic patient, then a series of diabetic patients and observed that the surgery seemed to reverse the disease process in 80-90% of their patients. The patients came in on insulin and, left a few days later off of it, perhaps never needing it again. Long before any weight loss occurred.

Dr. Francesco Rubino, who regaled the audience at the 2009 ADA meeting with his tales of rat bypass surgery, showed that type 2 diabetes seems to depend on specific food-gut interactions. He explained that a bypass works by separating a large portion of the stomach and rerouting the intestine so that food goes from a smaller stomach directly into the jejunum and passes through to the end of the small intestine. This "bypasses" most of the area where our digestion occurs. It helps with weight loss for obvious reasons: Your stomach is tiny, so you feel full quickly, and if you eat, it's hard to absorb the nutrients, since the small intestine has been bypassed. No intestine is actually removed in the process; it is just a re-arrangement of the anatomy with an end-result that can be diagramed as looking like a "Y":

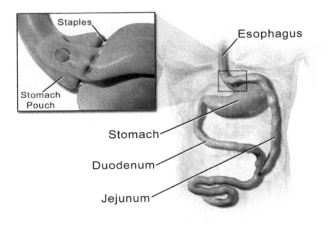

**Roux-En-Y**

*Source: wikicommons:wikimedia.org/Blausen 0776 Roux-En-Y 01.png*

Dr. Rubino performed bypass on rats bred to be obese and diabetic and showed that, just as in humans, type 2 diabetes went into remission with surgery. He then reversed the gastric bypass and showed that the diabetes came back. He postulated that the bypass, by depriving the small intestine of nutrients, was causing a change in the food-gut-hormone pathways that regulate how we deal with food energy.

To test this, he stuck tubes down the rats' throats through the stomach, past the first part of the intestine and found that it worked just like bypass: diabetes went away, without the big surgery. He pulled the tube out and the diabetes came back. He wanted to make sure that it wasn't just the tube doing something, so he put holes in the tube, so that food could leak out. The diabetes came back. Back and forth, over and over again, in these (he called them) heroic rats, with diabetes getting switched on and off, depending upon whether nutrients came in contact with the small intestine.

Today, these results have been reproduced everywhere that bariatric surgery is systematically studied. Gastric bypass as a "cure" for diabetes is commonplace (though many non-surgeon physicians seem not to know it). However, the results seem to vary by the method of surgery. If one compares gastric bypass to gastric banding (in which the stomach is constricted by the band into a small pouch similar to bypass, but is otherwise left intact) the banding patients do not have nearly half the luck regarding diabetes resolution, and it happens more slowly, apparently secondary to the weight loss. This would seem to make it obvious that Dr. Rubino and others were right when they considered diabetes to be caused by the interaction of nutrients with the duodenum (the first part of the intestine).

However, gastric "sleeve" bypass, which cuts away a lot of tissue, leaving only a sleeve shaped stomach to receive food, but without bypassing the duodenum, does almost as well as the traditional "Roux-En-Y" bypass. Logically, the sleeve bypass, which leaves one hooked up end to end without disruption, should do no better than banding if the cause of diabetes is simply food touching the duodenum. To examine this question further, Erik Hansen and colleagues looked at different routes of feeding and the effects this would have on hormonal responses to bypass surgery. Their goal was to test whether the food actually touching the duodenum was the direct cause of diabetes remission in bypass patients. They came up with a clever way to examine this hypothesis. They checked patients before and after bypass with regard to blood sugar, insulin and other related hormones. They checked how the patients' bodies reacted to food delivered to different parts of the digestive system by inserting a tube into the stomach, connected through the skin to the outside world, at the time of surgery.

This way, after surgery, the study subjects could eat food by mouth, have it travel down the bypass route straight to the jejunum (missing the duodenum), or have food put into the gastric tube connected to the stomach left after surgery (note in the diagram above, that the stomach remains in the body after Roux-En-Y bypass). This second way of feeding would put the food through the old route of: stomach, then duodenum, etc. So the subjects could act as their own controls in an experiment that compared a human reaction to the same food delivered in three ways: before surgery with normal anatomy, after surgery using bypassed anatomy and after surgery using a tube that would still have food pass through the entire small intestine (which is not removed during bypass, as it is needed to transport bile from the liver and digestive enzymes from the pancreas). What did they find?

For those of us who thought Dr. Rubino's rat experiments explained type 2 diabetes, as I did, the results were surprising. The patients all had improvements in blood sugar, insulin secretion, insulin sensitivity and other hormone response to food. But the route of food administered to the subjects *made no difference.* Whether food came into the stomach and touched the duodenum, or was eaten to bypass the duodenum, the patients appeared to be sensitive to insulin again. This argues that *something else* happens during or shortly after bariatric surgery to cause the change in insulin sensitivity. The surgery itself changed the way the subjects responded to food later, regardless of whether or not the food touched the duodenum, so we must conclude that there are other mechanisms at work.

In 2012, two papers in the *New England Journal of Medicine* made headlines for reporting diabetes remission rates between 37% and 95% with bariatric surgery (Schauer and colleagues, Mingrone and colleagues, both on 3/29/12). Previous accounts of diabetes remission after bypass were primarily observational. That is, they simply reported the outcomes for the patients that they operated on. They were without randomization and comparison groups. Based on those earlier studies, the consensus had been that type 2 diabetes is reversible by surgery with the following caveats:

—The shorter the duration of diabetes, the better.

—The milder the case, the better.

—Patients on insulin are harder to "cure."

—The more drastic the surgery, the better.

—Roux -En-Y is best for diabetes, then gastric sleeve, then gastric banding.

The *New England Journal* studies improve upon our understanding of these questions by comparing the surgery patients to conventional medical treatment groups. Both studies were able to quantify the degree of improvement expected by surgery, which previously was described qualitatively. The Schauer study was conservative in its conclusions, I think to a fault. By reporting the percentage of patients reaching a target hemoglobin A1C (a measure of average blood sugar over months) of less than 6% as the definition of remission of diabetes, they downplay the fact that the vast majority of surgery patients had tremendous improvement, stopped nearly all medications and came very close to complete remission at one year. The 37% and 42% remission reported tends to understate that improvement. The tables included in the article make clear that doctors can explain to patients with confidence that surgery will drastically improve diabetes, probably make all medicines unnecessary, and nearly guarantee a major change in the risk of long term complications such as heart disease and renal failure.

The trouble with both of the 2012 *New England Journal* studies is that the comparison group was "conventional medical therapy" (despite the fact that Schauer and colleagues termed it "intensive"). What does conventional medical therapy mean? This means piling one medicine on top of another to reach blood sugar targets and to give half-hearted advice about lifestyle changes. What do I mean by "half-hearted"? How about, "encouraged to participate in the Weight Watchers program"? To me, that's about as half-hearted as it gets. The diet advice was perhaps just slightly worse than what you might get from your neighbor . . . In my clinical experience, very few candidates for bariatric surgery have not tried Weight Watchers or other commercial programs, repeatedly.

## Surgery vs. Starvation

So, what would be a good non-surgical comparison group to test the mechanism of bariatric surgery's effect on diabetes? In a study published in 2011, E.L. Lim and colleagues tested whether eating like a bariatric surgery patient would have the same effect as actually having the surgery. In short: They starved their patients without first operating. This was set up to test what exactly needs to happen for diabetes to disappear. Is it the nerves that get cut or hormonal changes that occur with the operation? Is it altering the food/gut interaction? Could it simply be that you never eat much again?

They took 11 volunteers (people don't line up for starvation studies) with type 2 diabetes and fed them a diet of 600 calories per day for eight weeks. They found that after one week of dramatically reduced caloric intake, blood glucose levels entirely normalized in these diabetic patients. They also showed over the eight week study period that fatty liver and fatty pancreas (one of the keys to type 2 pathology) were entirely resolved. The patients were secreting a normal amount of insulin and their insulin resistance resolved as well. It was as if the patients had had surgery. Keep in mind that this was one hundred-year-old news when it came out. The original treatment of diabetes, both types, was starvation and/or complete carbohydrate restriction.

Is this a fair comparison? Starvation vs. bariatric surgery? It's a better comparison than "conventional medical therapy." I've worked in the bariatric surgeon's office and compared notes with the surgery dietitian. We've shared pictures of the meals eaten by successful surgery patients and successful weight loss patients in my clinic. Believe me, successful bariatric surgery patients are eating very little, perhaps not much more than the starvation patients in the Lim study. When surgery patients, over time, increase calories one, five, or ten years out, the weight begins to creep back. When surgery patients are in their first year of recovery and the weight is coming off effortlessly, they don't seem to regain a normal metabolism so much as they seem to be able to successfully follow a crazy rigid diet without any hunger. It makes them, to my mind, wired like a naturally skinny person: easily full, kind of nauseous with overeating and prone to eat more nutritive foods. Perhaps there is no mystery as to why the surgeries, such as gastric sleeve, which leaves the anatomy intact, are still quite useful for diabetes. Because of the surgery, food is drastically reduced. In addition, to avoid protein starvation, post-surgery patients are counseled (almost hounded) by the team's dietitians to meet protein goals before all else. It may actually be one of the highest protein and lowest carb diet programs out there.

With regard to long term follow up, surgery remains the most effective treatment we have for diabetes. However, medical physicians are generally reluctant to recommend this drastic approach to a disease that can be managed with medications. In addition, every physician has patients or knows of cases who have had the surgery and found only temporary relief of obesity and diabetes. These exceptions to the rule tend to make an impression, as they confirm our reasonable bias against invasive surgery. This is made worse by the track record of early surgical programs which took the heaviest, sickest patients for bypass first and, not surprisingly, had poor outcomes, including high mortality rates.

Since best practices and quality standards became widespread between 2000 and 2010, the mortality and other complications from gastric bypass have plummeted and the safety concerns are inaccurate. An analysis from Justin Dimick and colleagues published in *JAMA* in 2013 showed the mortality risk from gastric bypass to be equivalent to that of removing a gallbladder. It is possible that our reluctance to consider gastric bypass in our patients reflects an ongoing unconscious fat bias and an old-fashioned understanding of the disease: that it is caused by gluttony and can be cured by willpower. Once we drop this way of thinking, we should look for the most effective treatment available for our patients.

With the "sleeve" gastric bypass, there is nothing particularly "drastic" about the procedure. The operation takes less than one hour, it is performed through scope incisions, and blood loss is generally negligible. Yet physicians remain skeptical, pointing to the few exceptions they've seen. When I discuss this with patients, I point out that we don't stop sending people for knee replacement because we know of one or two patients who continued to experience pain, or needed re-operation, or even had blood clots and died. We consider these unfortunate outcomes as the rare, but possible, risks of any major surgery and believe that the benefits outweigh the risks. With regard to bariatric surgery, the irony is that we do continue to refer those same patients for knee replacements and other procedures with worse risk profiles than gastric bypass. We are only reluctant to send them for the one procedure that might lower their long term risks for bad outcomes from *any* procedure. The early operations didn't kill patients because the surgery was risky. It was risky to operate on those patients *for any reason*. The improvement in mortality that has occurred over the last 20 years reflects, in large part, surgeons selecting safer patients to operate on, rather than improvement in the surgical techniques.

In addition to a primary physician's lack of updated knowledge regarding the risks of bariatric surgery, there is the (again, unfounded) belief that the improvement in weight and diabetes with bariatric surgery is temporary. After five or ten years, some physicians believe, the diabetes comes right back. To assess this question, David Arterburn and colleagues followed over 4,000 gastric bypass patients for 10 years to look at the longer term results. Their study, published in *Obesity Surgery* in 2013, found 68% of previously diabetic bypass patients to be diabetes-free at 5 years and 40% to remain so at 10 years. To my way of thinking, this is a report of one of the major triumphs in modern medicine. While surgery can't be thought of as a universal cure for diabetes, after surgery, most medications, most especially injections with insulin, will be unnecessary, and the disease will almost certainly become easily managed with much lower long term health risk.

Lest we get too enthusiastic about a surgical cure, there are some important caveats to consider: First, while the mortality rate of bypass surgery has been dramatically reduced, there are still post-operative risks that come with sudden weight loss, starvation type eating, and poor absorption of nutrients. After surgery, deficiencies in iron, albumin, calcium and vitamin D are commonplace (Ikramuddin 2015). Bariatric surgery patients require supplementation and lifelong monitoring of vitamin levels. When surgery is performed on individuals unable or unwilling to be vigilant about protein intake, this deficiency will cause muscle wasting and hair loss. Additionally, surgery patients never get to enjoy food in the same way. The surgery forces tiny, very frequent feedings that need to be followed without the normal call and response of hunger and satiety. The general recommendation is to never eat and drink at the same sitting, as the liquid fills the smaller stomach and does not allow enough food to be consumed. Alcohol is considered off limits because fast absorption makes its effects felt much more quickly and addictions are more common after the surgery. It is safe to say that you would not wish this method of treatment on someone if they had other choices.

Obesity and diabetes are not the same. When it comes to type 2 diabetes, I think it is fair to say that patients have some good choices. Starting Metformin early, adding other oral medications when and if glucose is not controlled, and utilizing newer injectable medications and insulin when required, provide a host of opportunities to keep type 2 diabetes from causing serious harm. Surgery should continue to be reserved for the cases when these measures fail. But those measures do fail, quite often. Either through lack of ability on the patient's part to stick to monitoring and strict medication adherence, or due to the severity of the disease, many type 2 diabetic patients go on to have amputations, heart attacks and kidney failure. This is largely unnecessary in the present era of bariatric surgery. Earlier consideration of surgery should prevent the majority of those secondary consequences.

At meetings for bariatric societies, it is commonly stated that less than one percent of individuals who could qualify for gastric bypass surgery are having the procedure done. "Qualify" would mean, in this case, that a person's BMI is over 40 (generally 100 pounds overweight) or that there is a BMI of greater than 35 with diabetes. If a person fits those criteria, society guidelines and insurance are in favor of surgery. If we take the one percent number at face value and consider next steps, where does that lead?

If we were to recognize that bariatric surgery is vastly under-utilized, misunderstood and much more effective at treating obesity and type 2 diabetes than anything else, we might consider trying to put a dent in the 99% of the population that's not having surgery. To make any real progress, we could advocate for developing 10 times as many bariatric surgery centers as we currently have. In Iowa, where I live, this would mean that, instead of 5 centers, we would have 50 . . . in more populous states the numbers would be proportionate, so that in big cities you would see 40-50 bariatric surgery centers competing to re-route your gut.

Even if this were feasible, we would then be treating only 10% of those who qualify for surgery with one of the versions of gastric bypass. 90% of the risk for kidney failure, heart attacks and amputation would remain. It goes without saying that we can't scale up another order of magnitude to 400-500 surgery centers competing in big cities. We will simply have to do something with the food to get in front of this problem. Bariatric surgery is very effective, but also immensely impractical. The side effect profile for the procedure, if it were a daily medicine would surely cause many to stop treatment. I don't think we are ever going to live in a world where bariatric surgery is commonplace. I think it's much more likely that the solution to type 2 diabetes and obesity will occur elsewhere.

## References:

Hansen, E, et. al. Role of the foregut in the early improvement in glucose tolerance and insulin sensitivity following Roux-en-Y gastric bypass surgery. *American Journal of Physiology* 2011, 300(5): G795-G802.

Schauer, PR, et. al. Bariatric surgery versus intensive medical therapy in obese patients with diabetes. *NEJM* 2012, 366: 2567-2576.

Mingrone, G. et. al. Bariatric surgery versus conventional medical therapy for type 2 diabetes. *NEJM* 2012, 366: 1577-1585.

Lim, EL, et. al. Reversal of Type 2 Diabetes: normalization of beta cell function in association with decreased pancreas and liver triacylglycerol. *Diebetologia* 2011, 54(10): 2506-2014.

Dimick JB, et. al. Bariatric surgery complications before vs. after a national policy restricting coverage to Centers of Excellence. *JAMA* 2013, 309(8): 729-799.

Artenburn, DE. A multisite study of long-term remission and relapse of type 2 diabetes mellitus following gastric bypass. *Obesity Surgery* 2013, 23(1): 93-102.

Ikramuddin, S, et. al. Roux-En-Y gastric bypass for diabetes (the Diabetes Surgery Study): 2-year outcomes of a 5-year, randomized, controlled trial. *Lancet Diabetes Endocrinology* 2015, 3(6): 413-422.

# Chapter 6

## What Is Fat For?

Working as an occupational medicine physician in 2003, I became interested in metabolic syndrome. I was receiving an increasing number of requests coming from corporate clients to address the rise of obesity and diabetes in the workforce. Human resource directors, wellness teams and CEOs were keenly aware that the health costs of their employees were driven more by lifestyle factors than anything else, and I thought I might be able to help. Using the Diabetes Prevention Program as a model, I pitched and implemented a "metabolic clinic" for one of my client companies which performed yearly blood tests and wellness screens.

My longer term plan was to figure out which techniques of healthy eating would improve weight and blood sugar in a "high risk" pilot group and if successful, implement the program for the whole company in the following years. Assuming this worked, we could then roll out the program to other companies, modifying the program as we learned better how to control the factors that drive health risk and cost. I had initially considered addressing obesity directly as it had become a personal interest of mine, but there was a problem with trying to tackle obesity directly. This was that obesity is known to be a very *indirect* measure of health status acting over long periods of time. Knowing that obesity was both difficult to treat and slow to manifest measurable outcomes in terms of health cost, I proposed that we focus on lifestyle issues in those at highest risk of metabolic problems: workers whose blood sugar had already risen to a high borderline level. If we could arrest or reverse the signs of impending diabetes in this group, it would likely show obvious early health benefits and cost savings for the company. This would come through fewer doctor visits and prescription medications . . . perhaps we'd even avoid some heart attacks. We started with the borderline glucose group, then we sent invitations to anyone in the company whose wellness panel showed two more additional risk factors: obesity, low HDL cholesterol, high triglycerides, or high blood pressure. 20 individuals signed up and we soon began our pilot with the help of a dietitian and an athletic trainer.

My surprise came on the first day of clinic: None of the clients were very heavy. We counseled 10 people on diabetes risk, exercise and diet who didn't appear to weigh any more than the professionals counseling them. The second day of clinic came and went . . . and still, only a couple individuals had a clinically meaningful weight issue to discuss. Confused, I reviewed the data and our methods of choosing our candidates and realized something important in the database of the entire screened population: Weight and blood sugar didn't correlate very well. I ran calculations looking for BMI's effect on blood sugar in excel and there simply was no relationship:

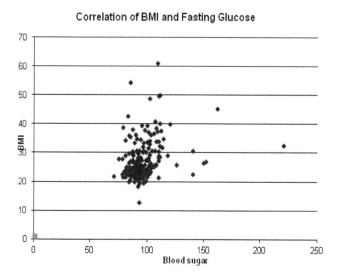

**Correlation of BMI and Fasting Glucose**

*If there was a positive correlation between higher BMIs and higher fasting glucose, you would see a graph looking more like a line, heading up and out to the right. This instead shows the classic "blob" that designates no correlation between the variables whatsoever.*

This ran contrary to how I had learned about these illnesses, but I soon realized what was going on: By focusing on glucose in a young healthy working group, we were pulling out the most metabolically susceptible individuals, who were not necessarily those that had become obese . . . yet.

I realized that the correlation between obesity and diabetes that is often reported in large cross-sectional surveys doesn't tell us anything about the sequence of events, or about cause and effect. I had always assumed that people first over-ate, then became obese, then too much fat tissue made them insulin resistant, and if they went on getting heavier, they would eventually meet full criteria for diabetes. This pilot group we selected as high risk for diabetes showed me that it doesn't happen in that order. The people I was working with were both "pre-diabetic" and "pre-obese." The two diseases were coming on in parallel, due to some other factor . . . call it "X."

When I was in medical school in the 1990s, we still called it "Syndrome X." The syndrome was conceptualized and described by Gerald Reaven, a Stanford endocrinologist doing laboratory research on lipids, who gave a ground breaking lecture at an American Diabetes Association meeting in 1988. In that lecture, he laid out his two decades of incremental accumulation of evidence that insulin resistance was responsible for as many, if not more, heart attacks as high LDL cholesterol. He argued that his lab and many others had shown that high triglycerides in the blood, along with poor tolerance to glucose, low HDL cholesterol, and hypertension were all mediated by insulin. These factors, he argued, caused the 50% of heart attacks that could not be explained by the high cholesterol model and perhaps suggested an alternate way of looking at why coronary artery disease and strokes occur.

Why he chose to name it "Syndrome X" as if the cause was unknown, rather than "the insulin resistance syndrome" is something I can't understand. I do know that in 1993, in my basic medical school lectures, when the idea was still working its way into the consciousness of researchers and clinicians, the name made it sound mysterious. We didn't think of insulin as having anything to do with fat handling and we were taught that obesity was a behavioral disorder (one that we didn't spend much time on, as a matter of fact). The Syndrome X nomenclature seemed to hide the point that insulin resistance was the missing factor that doctors were not seeing.

A decade later, as I puzzled over what to do with my "pre-obese" clients who were showing signs of all the metabolic abnormalities described by Reaven, the cluster of findings had since been re-named to "metabolic syndrome." But that still didn't help me know what to do next. Was there a diet and exercise program that directly addressed the cause of metabolic syndrome? Calling it "insulin resistance syndrome," wouldn't have made it any easier for me to proceed. The question was: Why were people becoming insulin resistant in the first place? Insulin resistance wasn't an ultimate cause, but a marker and an expression of something else. I got to work reading the papers published by Reaven and others.

As the idea of "low-carb" dieting was beginning another trendy phase at that time, I was surprised to see that Dr. Reaven had been cautioning against low-fat diets since the mid-sixties, contending that they were unlikely to help LDL and very likely to cause worsening triglycerides and blood sugar. He had warned in the early 1980s that universal adoption of low-fat diets was a mistake and bound to harm some of those for whom LDL was never a problem. He seemed like a prophet when I read him in 2003, but more importantly, his papers and those of researchers who followed his reasoning, showed me what was happening in my clients' bodies. The following is my summary of his teaching.

There are three different metabolic scenarios: One type of person is normal, with blood pressure under control, LDL and HDL in the normal range, triglycerides normal, and blood sugar normal. This is the most common finding of any group you would usually screen at a yearly company wellness drive. The second scenario is the one your doctor is most familiar with: Most of the numbers are normal, but your LDL, or "bad" cholesterol is too high. This is easily remedied by taking Lipitor or any of the other "statin" drugs, which most doctors are quick to do. Treating LDL is one of the most common general medicine activities around and it's straight out of the traditional view that high cholesterol causes buildup of fat in the coronary arteries that eventually become big enough to stop blood flow and cause a heart attack. The third metabolic profile is actually pretty strange: Blood pressure is up, blood sugar is borderline high, triglycerides are high, LDL is normal and HDL, or "good" cholesterol is low. The LDL is actually "small and dense" in character, making it more likely to cause problems, but the number is normal on the lab test. This is the metabolic syndrome. Dr. Reaven showed that all of these happen in the context of insulin resistance with the most direct cause being a high carbohydrate diet. To understand why, we need to think about cholesterol in a little more detail.

LDL and all the rest are "lipoproteins." They are measurable globs of fatty stuff in our blood that can be separated and counted. The globs are of different sizes and densities. There are actually hundreds of different-sized globs of fat circulating in the blood, but we categorize them into families and we focus on the few for which we have a decent guess regarding their purpose in the body. The HDLs are "high density," and if you were to eyeball a test tube of human plasma, they'd be down near the bottom, because they are densest. The LDLs would rise to the top like cream, because they are "low density." What makes them light or dense, in the simplest sense, is whether they are full of fat and cholesterol or not. They also have different roles in moving lipids about. LDLs, in general, are heading out into the circulation, while HDLs are heading back to the liver. HDLs represent a particle that has capacity to pick up cholesterol molecules. If you eat too much, or make too much cholesterol, HDL can take it back to the liver and out of circulation before it deposits in your artery wall. LDLs are basically full of fat and cholesterol and they are about to disgorge it somewhere you probably do not want it.

Cholesterol science is confusing and the terminology doesn't do much to help. For starters, we call HDL and LDL "cholesterol," which isn't accurate. They *transport* cholesterol. Also, we call them "lipoproteins" but they really don't perform like proteins and aren't composed of amino acid chains like a protein. They are lipid droplets. They have proteins in their outer membranes that help them get absorbed into different tissues, but they really aren't proteins in any real sense. They are, as I say, best thought of as a bunch of globs floating around, carrying cholesterol and triglycerides.

We report a triglyceride number in the lab results along with HDL and LDL, but triglycerides are not actually a glob, like LDL or HDL, they are molecules, more like cholesterol itself, which isn't measured directly. They are something that is carried inside the lipoproteins, mostly VLDL (very low density lipoprotein)

117

and chylomicrons which come from the gut after we eat. LDL and HDL also carry some triglycerides, but mostly traffic in cholesterol.

So how do we account for the lipid profile of the patient with metabolic syndrome? Why don't they just have a high LDL like regular cardiac patients? What makes this a "syndrome"? To tie the various signs together into a syndrome, we need to consider how the body reacts to meals in the modern environment. Like most of us, those with metabolic syndrome are eating a high calorie, high-fat, high-carbohydrate diet (trust me, I review the diet logs). The carbohydrates we eat each meal break down to sugar, which goes to the liver. The liver says, in essence, "Good, I've got enough sugar for energy, I can get rid of these triglycerides I've been storing all day." So high triglycerides (fat in the blood) can be caused by carbohydrate in the diet. After a high-carb meal, the liver releases VLDL particles, full of triglycerides into the blood. Meanwhile, the fat that we eat is absorbed by the intestines and packaged into particles called chylomicrons. So, after eating a fat and carbohydrate rich meal, we have two reasons for high triglycerides: what we've absorbed directly from our meal and what's been put out from the liver.

Here's where it gets interesting: HDL and LDL, floating around in the blood stream, are able to exchange some of their contents (cholesterol molecules) with each other and also with chylomicrons and VLDL. This happens in low grade fashion all the time; it's just one of the numerous balancing acts the body uses to keep things regulated. However, this ability to exchange lipids between particles can be altered by our dietary habits. When there is a high number of VLDL from the liver (from eating too much carbohydrate) and a lot of chylomicrons (from eating too much fat), more exchange happens than would normally be expected. HDL and LDL give up some of their cholesterol in exchange for triglycerides, so they become "small and dense." The small HDLs go to the kidney, which takes them out of circulation. This makes our HDL number "low" when we measure it. The LDLs stay in the blood stream as "small and dense," but their overall number is normal (Barter 2006). The triglycerides are measured as high because the high-fat, high-sugar, high-calorie diet makes it high by the methods explained above.

This gives us the signature lipid panel of the metabolic syndrome patient: high triglycerides, low HDL, and normal (smaller, denser) LDL.

To consolidate the above: The particles are not unique, separate entities, but run a gamut of sizes from high density to very low, with all sizes in between as they morph and bump into each other, exchanging their contents via enzymes like cholesteryl ester transfer protein. Rather than separate entities, it would be simplest to think of them as different versions of the same protein (or "glob" of fat, really) that can present differing lipid panels when checked in the lab, *depending upon what we eat.* The high TG, low HDL, normal LDL profile is simply the human adaptation to a high-fat, high-carbohydrate diet. Notice that high triglycerides and borderline glucose are what you'd see if you did a *non-fasting* blood panel on nearly anyone. These things are *supposed to* go up if we've just eaten. What's different about our patients with the metabolic syndrome, is that the blood looks like it's in a "fed" state, even after an overnight fast. By and large, my metabolic syndrome patients are not breakfast eaters. Why? Because there's fuel sitting in the bloodstream already, in the form of a high fasting glucose and triglyceride, so their brain thinks they've been fed. Until the boom and bust of sugar feeding starts later in the day, my patients are relatively hunger free.

What I learned by focusing on my pre-diabetic, "pre-obese" population is that the constant refrain of physicians to their patients, "If you lost a little weight, all of these problems would improve," is actually inaccurate. It assumes that it is weight loss, itself, that causes improvement in the metabolic parameters. In fact, the weight, or more specifically, the increased adiposity, is a symptom, just as lower HDL and higher triglycerides are symptoms. Obesity improves as the other metabolic parameters improve and by the same method: improvement of poor nutrition habits. In the case of the metabolic syndrome clients, this means lowering fat and carbohydrate in the diet.

When we re-assessed the pre-diabetic workers who signed up to try diet and exercise for diabetes prevention, our results matched those of many trials. Weight loss correlated with improved blood glucose, a better "good/bad" cholesterol ratio and lower triglycerides. The measures moved in parallel, reversing the poor metabolism through diet and exercise. Just the diabetes prevention program outcomes had shown, very little weight loss was needed to improve metabolic syndrome in my group. This shows us that the human body is not waiting for a reduction in the fat stores before allowing the other markers of metabolic syndrome to improve. Food determines the markers, simultaneously, or even regardless of weight loss, because reducing the amount of fat on the body doesn't have anything to do with metabolic consequences. The fat itself, the adipose tissue on the body, is not the cause of metabolic syndrome, rather, *an adaptation to it.*

## Fat Is Useful

Roger Unger and Phillip Scherer are University of Texas researchers who argue that fat doesn't cause diabetes, but rather helps delay it. The role of the fat tissue, they explain, is to act as a cushion for excess energy we consume, not only so that we can use it later, but because it can be damaging to the other tissues of the body. While there are a host of behavioral explanations for why dieting doesn't work, these researchers argue that the most important factor limiting our ability to lose weight is that our body doesn't share our disdain for the adipose tissue. In fact, the body, the part we like, the muscles and other organs comprising the lean tissue, is quite dependent on fat's presence. Why? Drs Scherer and Unger believe (and have shown quite clearly in mice) that the fat cells act like an organ whose main purpose is to protect us against the ill effects of overeating. In a 2003 article provocatively titled "Weapons of Lean Body Mass Destruction: The Role of Ectopic Lipids in the Metabolic Syndrome" Dr. Unger shows how much worse off we would be without fat to protect us from our diets.

With the exception of fat tissue, he explains, no body organ does very well in the presence of fatty acids. If a body did not have the ability to store fat over time, the fat would infiltrate our muscles, liver, pancreas, heart and wreak havoc . . . which is what it actually does when the adipose tissue becomes poorly regulated. Dr. Unger points out that this is actually what "metabolic syndrome" is: our body having trouble coping with excess calories, which results in damage to the cells not specifically equipped to handle it. Why do the other tissues have trouble with fat? They lack some of the specialized enzymes that help package and process it. Any cells which receive more fat than is needed for immediate energy, allow those fatty acids to go through alternate metabolic pathways. Many of these lesser-used pathways lead to stress on the inner components of the cell. This sends off distress signals which sometimes result in the cells dying off.

Cell death in response to stress is one of our body's ways of dealing with toxins. The body needs to shut down the processes of cells that have gone awry in order to keep the other cells functioning well. So, when things get too out of balance (as in cancer, or infection) the body is pretty good at just killing off problem cells. This causes trouble in the context of overeating and the pancreas, because the fat we eat can get compartmentalized in the beta cells that make insulin. The excess fat derails the normal metabolism, the cells send off distress signals and then the beta cells begin to die off. This is the later stage type 2 diabetes: An inability to secrete enough insulin to process the carbohydrates that we eat, because the beta cells have been systematically destroyed in an effort to preserve function. This is a little bit different than our typical explanation for diabetes: first you eat too much, then you get fat, then that fat screws up your metabolism and makes you diabetic. In particular, the role of the fat cell, in the eyes of Unger and Scherer, is re-written from villain to hero. As they explain in an article published in *Trends in Endocrinology and Metabolism* (2010), the fat cells valiantly combat the ill effects of over-nutrition by expanding their activity, storing energy to protect the more sensitive pancreas, muscle and heart, which don't deal well with excess calories. The fat cells grow and multiply as a protective adaptation to how we are living. They are not the cause of diabetes, but rather, the *one thing* protecting us from it.

They refer to the process as "lipotoxicity." The fat that we eat can act like a toxin in our tissues. The fatty acids and triglycerides that are the product of taking in more energy than can be used or stored are harmful locally due to producing inflammatory signals that both damage cells and cause cell death. The lean, healthy body is one that is able to partition and traffic energy into the fat cells to be stored, or to muscles to be used for work. Individuals susceptible to metabolic disorders like diabetes are not as good at sending the fat to the right places and this helps drive the metabolic illnesses. The hormones leptin and adiponectin, both made in the fat cells, play key roles in this process. Leptin, which gets secreted in greater quantities as the fat cells grow, acts in a number of protective ways including serving as a "stop eating" baseline signal to the brain. Adiponectin has several roles as well. A key feature seems to be turning on each cell's machinery to effectively process fat, rather than letting it cause damage. The levels and balance of these hormones are likely variable between individuals, which yields a varying susceptibility to obesity and diabetes. Through describing the mechanisms of these hormones derived from the fatty tissue, Unger and

Scherer show us that fat is necessary and vital to our health.

## Do Dietary Carbohydrates Cause High Blood Sugar?

With regard to my metabolically at risk patients, the initial group did quite well with no new cases of diabetes in the first year, which was better than a comparison group made up of similar workers who chose not to participate. The numbers were too small to say definitively, but I came away convinced that very modest changes in diet could have dramatic effects on risk. As I moved on to work with more patients who had a chief complaint of obesity, it seemed that lower carbohydrate diets seemed to improve patient numbers the quickest. We didn't use carbohydrate elimination, resulting in ketosis, but simple lower-carb dieting with a focus on calorie counting to avoid overeating. However, there was a fair bit of variety in the results. Not all of my patients had good luck with a simple prescription of reducing carbohydrate to about 40% of intake. The diabetic patients, in particular, seemed to have more difficulty with low-carb advice and returned with glucose tracking logs that didn't match my simple theory very well. Their sugars were all over the map and I didn't know if it was because they were worse at following a lower-carb diet, or whether there was something in their actual metabolism that gave diabetic patients a different reaction. Eating carbs sustains the blood sugar. If we reduce carbs, we have to reduce blood sugar, don't we?

I decided to run an experiment on myself. The plan was to test the principles I was recommending to patients in my weight loss program (eat more protein, eat less carb, don't worry about fat) while measuring my blood sugar regularly. After a week, I would revert to my usual devil-may-care diet and count up the difference a few basic changes could make. The second week would, of course, show higher blood sugars, even though I'm healthy (especially since I would make a point of eating my sweets). I pictured being able to show some very clear slides at future obesity talks: Week one, behaving well —sugar is smooth. Week two, eat like an American —blood sugar high and erratic. If it worked well, I could also show this to new patients who were still reluctant to believe: "Look, this is a graph of my blood sugar with normal eating; look at the difference after I go low-carb—"

So what actually happened?

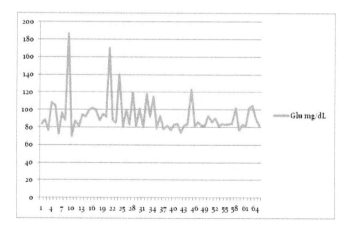

The above shows my blood sugars over what ended up being 12 days of testing. The values up until number 45 are the moderate- carb, higher protein diet and the glucose readings after 45 are what happened when I basically went nuts on sugar, eating Apple Jacks, candy canes, chocolate and drinking Coke (it was Christmas time). It's easy to see the pattern here. Notice how smooth and low the values are *after* the 45th reading, with almost no values peaking over 100. My average daily glucose was 95.9 mg/dL on the lower-carb diet and 85.6 mg/dL *on the higher-carb diet*. The average increase in glucose after meals the first week was 20.5 mg/dL and only 4.5 mg/dL the second. The controlled diet had much higher spikes in blood sugar than the indulgent, more typically "American" diet. Eating 500-1000 calories more and 100 extra grams of carbohydrate per day, I saw consistently *lower* blood sugars!

In the second week of the experiment, I got so frustrated at seeing such a steady stream of blood glucose values in the 80s that I began trying with all my might to make my blood glucose go up after meals by ingesting the worst garbage I could think of. One evening I drank three Coca-Colas in a row, while checking blood sugar every half hour . . . and reached a peak of only 95 mg/dL. A couple days later, I strutted into my coffee shop, determined to show my pancreas who's boss. I ordered a mocha and a chocolate croissant, then a second mocha and downed the whole 820 calories (with 116 grams of simple sugar) in 20 minutes, thinking, "Surely, if ever there was a meal that was created to provoke one's blood sugar, this is it." I then checked my glucose every 10 minutes to find the spike . . . which reached 105 mg/dL at 30 minutes before normalizing down to the 80s again. Then I stopped to think about how insulin works.

## How Insulin Works

In a healthy, non-diabetic, non-obese body, insulin is capable of handling doses of incoming calories and sugar without difficulty. Generally within an hour, certainly two, a healthy body will achieve a normal glucose level of less than 100, regardless of the meal. Insulin is secreted in two phases. The first phase happens when sweets hit the tongue. The pancreas knows that sugar is coming, so releases a bunch of insulin that is pre-packaged in little packets that are sent into the blood stream. Insulin begins immediately shuttling the glucose out of the blood and into the liver, muscles and fat cells. It then turns on the machinery to make more insulin from scratch, depending upon how much glucose has entered the blood during the meal. A second wave of insulin that was made in response to the particular meal gets released over 30 to 60 minutes, bringing the blood sugar down to a normal level by hour two, at latest. This is why many of the tests for diabetes check glucose two hours after a known load of sugar. The first phase of insulin secretion doesn't get turned on much by protein or fat, it is responding to the sugar content in the meal. Thus, sugary foods actually turn on the insulin mechanism *better* than protein or fat, which can drive the blood sugar lower (in some individuals) after a high-carb meal than a lower carb meal. Sugar and insulin are in balance and in tune with each other.

127

This way of thinking works for a healthy body. Granted, this was a crude experiment, run on one free-living individual, using finger-stick glucose measures, but it is evidence that we need to think twice about giving generic diet advice regarding carbohydrates. A more important question than how one healthy individual's blood sugars look over 12 days is how does this look in those whose insulin doesn't respond so well? How does all this play out in type 2 diabetic patients?

In "A Low-Carbohydrate, Ketogenic Diet to Treat Type 2 Diabetes," William Yancy and colleagues ran a more professional version of my home-grown experiment. Instead of focusing on the post-meal blood sugars, they waited a full three months to see how the blood glucose would average out in terms of hemoglobin A1C (a measure of how well one's blood sugar is controlled over longer periods). They found that a very low-carbohydrate diet (under 50 grams per day) lowered the average A1C by 16% even while medications were reduced or stopped in the majority of the participants. Their conclusion was that a low-carbohydrate diet was more effective than traditional (low-fat) diet counseling for the long term control of blood sugar in diabetic patients.

One hypothesis for reconciling the conflicting results of my brief experiment with the more formal study above is that I don't know what I'm doing. Another might be that non-diabetic bodies react to sugar and complex carbohydrates differently than diabetic bodies. What is diabetes but an inability to handle carbohydrate exposure? But just because the main feature of the disease is high blood sugar after ingesting carbohydrates, we cannot assume that carbohydrates *cause* the disease.

That's as silly as thinking that eating cholesterol causes heart disease, just because some people with heart disease have high cholesterol in the blood. In both cases, we are mistaking a symptom, or sign, with the cause of the disease. The problem in diabetes is poor blood sugar *regulation,* not simply sugar *ingestion.*

In "Continuous Glucose Profiles in Healthy Subjects under Everyday Life Conditions and after Different Meals," G. Freckmann and colleagues used continuous glucose monitors to check the response of healthy adults to different foods. Like me, they used mixed meals containing more or less carbohydrate, protein and fat. But unlike me, they got very accurate blood sugar numbers using continuous glucose monitors, which track blood sugar every five minutes. Also, unlike me, they found that the blood sugars of the participants responded exactly as biology would predict: Higher protein, higher fiber meals had smaller and slower increases in glucose than higher carb, low-fiber, low-protein meals.

The blood sugar responses in this study seemed to be more closely associated with the *percentage* of carbohydrates in a meal than the *quantity.* In fact, they kept the amount of carbohydrates in the test meals essentially constant at 50 grams per meal. Fiber seemed to be the best determinant of blood sugar control (my interpretation, looking at their tables) with protein percent and fat percent close behind. The highest fiber, highest protein meals had less than half the increase in blood sugar than the lowest fiber, lowest protein meals. However, the ranges of response were very wide, to the extent that there may have been individuals who reacted exactly opposite to the general trend (someone like me,

129

perhaps). This is why actual studies are superior to checking your own glucose in the coffee shop: The average results of a group are much more likely to give logical, true results than individual cases, especially over short periods of investigation.

One surprising feature of the results in this study is that calories (just as I had seen in my body) did not seem to matter. The meal which produced the smallest area under the curve for glucose was 16.5% protein, 26.8% carbohydrate (1/4th of this was fiber), 56.7% fat and 750 calories. The meal with the greatest area under the curve was 14.2% protein, 74.6% carbohydrate (no fiber), 11.2% fat and only 271 calories . . . same amount of carbs remember, just mixed to a lesser degree with protein, fat and fiber. Essentially, the more dilute and hidden the carbs in the meal (given the same *quantity* of carbs) the lower the blood sugar. It was not a trivial difference: On the high percentage carbohydrate meal, blood sugar peaked at 133.2 mg/dL. On the low percentage carb meal it reached an average of only 99.2 mg/dL. This is essentially the difference between healthy and unhealthy.

Note that fat is either an innocent bystander to the whole process, or it contributes to lower blood sugar based on these results. They didn't test that and I don't want to speculate. But, it must be pointed out that the traditional advice given to diabetic patients, to eat a low-fat diet, has no backing from this small data set.

So, why, considering all this, do dietitians and the endocrinologists who treat diabetes most typically recommend low-fat, traditional "heart protective" diets rather than lower carbohydrate? The most obvious answer is that they are not actually "considering all this."

A current specialist in diabetes has been trained in a school of thought codified in textbooks which have changed little since the 1990s. If they are paying attention at all, they are probably wondering why their advice fails to achieve good results most of the time. The recent trend has been to do less and less diet teaching and get type 2 diabetic patients on insulin sooner rather than later. Many of the most up-to-date dietitians and nurses certified as diabetes educators have chucked trying to manage diet at all and have become experts in adjusting insulin instead. Can you blame them? We know diets almost always fail in the end.

## References:

Diabetes Prevention Program Research Group. *NEJM* 2002, 346: 393-403.

Reaven, GM. Banting lecture 1988: Role of insulin resistance in human disease. *Diabetes* 1988, 37(12): 1595-607.

Reaven, Gerald. *Syndrome X: Overcoming the Silent Killer That Can Give You a Heart Attack.* New York: Simon and Schuster 2000.

Barter, PJ and Kastelein, JJ. Targeting cholesteryl ester transfer protein for the prevention and management of cardiovascular disease. *Journal of the American College of Cardiology* 2006, 47(3): 492-499.

Unger, RH and Scherer, PE. Gluttony, sloth and the metabolic syndrome: a roadmap to lipotoxicity. *Trends in Endocrinology and Metabolism* 2010, 21(6): 343-52.

Unger, RH. Minireview: weapons of lean body mass destruction: the role of ectopic lipids in the metabolic syndrome. *Endocrinology* 2003, 14(12): 5159-65.

Yancy, WS. et. al. A low-carbohydrate, ketogenic diet to treat type 2 diabetes. *Nutrition and Metabolism* 2005, 2:34.

Freckmann, G. et. al. Continuous glucose profiles in healthy subjects under everyday life conditions and after different meals. *Journal of Diabetes Science and Technology* 2007, 1(5): 695-703.

# Chapter 7

# Promise and Perils of High Protein

The realization that everything would be okay regarding the obesity epidemic occurred to me in a doughnut shop. It was the last week of my employment as a weight loss doctor, and for years, my clinic had been a junk food-free zone. This was not because I set rules based on a notion that junk food is bad for a person. I didn't and I don't really have much worry about occasional sugary snacks. It just happened as a sort of accidental byproduct of what we were doing. If you talk about diet rules all day and see how hard patients are working to eat better, it just feels wrong to have a big box of doughnuts in the break-room . . . or powdered sugar on your slacks.

So, there I was in Dunkin' Donuts to pick up a dozen fatty sugar bombs as an ironic goodbye gesture for my co-workers. When I got to the counter, at the register, I saw what was on display for an impulse buy: a Dunkin' Donuts protein bar.

As Austin Powers said, *"Yay! Capitalism!"*

Here, in the symbolic heart of the environmental disruption of our food supply was the beginning of the end of obesity. Actually, my very first thought was, "These people will do anything for money."

I believe that the future shows signs of being a healthier place for us, not by restricting choice or technology, but by using those two things to our biological and social advantage. What's occurring on the television, online, and in the grocery store tells us much about where we are going. Take Nature Valley granola bars, for instance. I have been pointing out this brand to my patients for years as an example of a company projecting an image of health for marketing purposes without any knowledge or concern about what makes a person healthy. The ingredients on a granola bar are fine; they won't hurt you, but they aren't suitable for people watching their weight. It's essentially a candy bar for people who can't admit to themselves that they want a candy bar. In any case, instead of broadcasting that the bar is made with whole grain, or is low-fat, as in past years, the new label broadcasts: Protein.

This, in fact, represents a change in the bar's recipe. The company spotted the protein trend, likely asked their target demographic what they are looking for in a healthy snack, and put it in the bars. Whole grain oats last decade, protein this decade, as long as it sells. It doesn't matter whether the company is doing it for ethical reasons, health reasons, or financial reasons. It also doesn't matter if the consumer is seeking foods with protein broadcast on the label because they are dieting, weight lifting, following paleo, Atkins, protein power, or have read Gary Taubes. It doesn't matter if people are even doing it deliberately at all. Trends occur for a multitude of reasons, but the need for profit ensures that companies listen, eventually, to their consumers. About 20 years into the espresso drink trend, even McDonald's picked up on the fact that it might be smart to try something different with its coffee. Thus we find hope for the modern world.

When I finally got to start a weight loss clinic (after asking my employers for years) in 2011, one of my most common discussions with patients was "how to find protein." At that point in time, in the Midwest anyway, convenience stores and grocery stores were not yet aware that these products were important. At our local grocery chain, a couple of brands of protein powder were kept in the functional food section of the store. Right next to Pedialyte and Ensure, you could pick up protein powder marketed as a muscle builder for weight lifters. That's what people in 2011 thought protein was for. It was a food that was semi-medicinal, available right near the pharmacy. Now, protein has become its own food group. Just as the grocery aisles highlight important items that are available in that row, such as "pasta" or "paper products," you can now find a label for "protein" in our local CVS. In the "protein aisle" are a host of bars (what we used to call energy bars, when we wanted energy, but now call protein bars), powders, cookies and even "protein water." Quaker Oats now makes a high-protein oatmeal. This is likely a response to consumers, who used to go through the trouble of adding protein powder to the oatmeal themselves. Cold breakfast cereals, as well, now increasingly include higher protein versions of our favorites.

Even Coca-Cola now sells protein. In 2014, as part of its ongoing mission to save the world from obesity (or maybe they wanted to make money, it's always hard to tell with the folks at Coke), the company purchased Core Power, which makes widely available shakes which I used to recommend to patients. Core Power took the consumer's desire for protein and married it to the consumer's interest in "real" ingredients and marketed their shakes as more "natural" than other brands. Instead of adding in amino acids from another food industry process (such as cheese making) the Core Power people hyper-filter cow's milk until it contains more protein and less carbohydrate. This gives them substantially fewer ingredients on the label, which consumers take as a sign of a better, purer, healthier product.

This worked so well that Coca-Cola noticed them, bought them and began making a high protein milk called Fairlife, which has twice the protein and one half the carbohydrate of regular milk (at twice the price). I like it, but then again, I like milk just fine and drink a ton of it for an adult (I also drink a ton of Coke for an adult, truth be told). Is Coca-Cola pushing protein a good thing? From an obesity doctor perspective, it's a great thing. People will consume what's displayed in the grocery store, or placed on the counter at the doughnut shop. If they don't, those things will not be there for long (Yay, Capitalism, once more). The Coca-Cola Company is good at spreading what it sells, opening up new markets and influencing what goes into our bodies. It might be argued that the more Coca-Cola gets involved in selling the protein trend, the better for our weight. The fact that protein is the buzz word for corporations and food marketers at this point in time likely bodes well for our obesity problem.

Protein is now on the cover of the package. It's getting top billing for once. This represents a new public consensus that we are leaving the era of fat, cholesterol and sugar concern and entering a new one: a period where people consciously seek protein. The protein leverage hypothesis argues that we have been unconsciously seeking it all along, but we can now align what little of our eating is controlled by the decision-making part of the brain with the unconscious needs of the body. To the extent that the "food industry" has been a willing or unwilling accomplice to the obesity epidemic, it will now (not because of intelligence or moral rectitude, but by the mechanisms inherent in capitalism) work against the obesity trend through the math of protein leverage. The more protein available, advertised, marketed, and displayed by companies with which we are already familiar, the more we will consume.

There is some irony in the big agribusiness and food production giants increasing protein in their products and charging us for the improvement. As an occupational medicine doctor in Cedar Rapids, Iowa, I had the lucky experience of touring the plants responsible for almost every aspect of turning rows of corn and wheat from the fields into foods which can be boxed and shipped and stored for several months and still taste wonderful. In our Midwestern city, we have a system of railways which would make Dr. Seuss or Rube Goldberg proud in its complexity. Corn, oats and wheat arrive on rail-cars from all over the continent. Cargill, ADM, General Mills, Quaker Oats and a variety of smaller plants, cooperate to rip these grains apart for every bit of sellable energy or chemical power they contain. I picture this whole complicated operation having now to fit reverse switches on several of the rails and pipes. After all the trouble taken to remove the hard nutritious bit to make wheat germ and save the yummy carbs for rolling into Wheaties flakes, the customer now wants the protein added back in!

It was John Harvey Kellogg in Battle Creek (The doctor's brother, William K., became the cereal maker) who convinced the country to eat a high-carbohydrate breakfast for our health (and for the health of the pigs and chickens he didn't think we should disturb). But now, *Special K* is one of the proudest promoters of protein-enhanced cereals, bars and shakes (Incidentally, they've done a better job putting the word "protein" on their packaging, than they have putting the stuff in the actual products . . . their protein shakes have the same content as milk). It seems strange for companies to do all this processing gymnastics just to bring back the breakfast macronutrient balance we had 150 years ago. Bacon, eggs and toast seems a well-designed combo to me.

The math of protein leverage estimates that as you increase protein percent in the diet, calories will decrease —about 100-200 calories per 5%, was my observation from patient journals. Even before I had discovered the scientific explanation, my patients and I seemed to have hit upon a solid solution for the obesity problem: just add protein. I took this notion to heart so deeply that my standard advice to anyone asking me about weight loss became: Just drink a protein shake a day for the next few months and see what happens.

What would be the ramifications if this advice became the common wisdom? What if the population became convinced that protein was the solution to weight problems and began to consume 25 or 30 extra grams in the morning, as I've advocated to all of my patients? Combine a greater protein awareness among the public and the food giants' willingness to supply us, and we may be about to find out. Simpson and Raubenheimer, the developers of the Protein Leverage hypothesis, have some thoughts on this:

*"Perhaps, then, augmenting the proportion of protein in the daily diet offers a means of ameliorating obesity by taking advantage of the inhibition of intake once the protein target is reached. Three things take some of the gloss from this optimistic suggestion."* —The Nature of Nutrition, page 185

They proceed to elaborate on the three hesitations: 1) it might not work, 2) it would be bad for the environment to increase livestock for our consumption, but most importantly, 3) more protein may actually be worse for human health. This last objection would be a cruel irony. We all shift our consumption to match the latest health consensus, that high protein is better than other diets, only to find out that it causes unintended health problems that are worse than the ones we are trying to avoid (Does this sound familiar?).

The environmental issues can be considered outside the scope of the present discussion. But the concerns regarding any risks of increased dietary protein are critical to our discussion. Simpson and Raubenheimer reiterated their caution regarding the use of high protein as a diet strategy in a more recent paper that appeared in *Cell:*

*"A major conclusion from the geometric experiments on flies and mice is that the balance of macronutrients in the diet has a profound impact on food and energy*

*intake, metabolic health, lifespan, immune function and reproduction. The diet composition that best supports longevity is not the same as that which sustains maximal reproductive output or leanness." —Simpson, et. al. 2015.*

**Too Much of a Good Thing?**

There are only three macronutrients in the diet. Have scientists, in addition to looking at the consequences of high-carb diets and high-fat diets, looked at the health consequences of high-protein diets?

Luckily for our current discussion, they have. Regarding the efficacy of higher protein diets for weight loss, many trials and reviews have corroborated the principle of protein leverage by testing higher versus lower protein diets while controlling the carbohydrate and fat eaten. For example, in 2005, David Weigle and colleagues published a trial comparing diets of equal calories that contained either normal, or twice normal protein (15% and 30% respectively). The authors point out, in their introduction, that low-carb diets (which are high fat) and low-fat diets seem to work equally well and that our current thinking requires dietary fat to make fat in our bodies. "This paradox could be explained if it is the high protein content, rather than the lower carbohydrate content of low-carbohydrate diets that offsets the deleterious effect of high fat intakes and results in weight loss."

The researchers assessed baseline calorie needs, metabolism and a variety of hormone levels during two weeks in which the subjects were fed diets of 15%

protein, 50% carbohydrate, and 35% fat (the usual diet considered U.S. standard). After two weeks of this, the researchers doubled the protein to 30% but required the subjects to eat all of the food provided, which kept calories the same. Eating higher protein at the same calorie level did *not* produce weight loss, although the subjects rated hunger much lower and fullness much higher during the double protein period. Dr. Weigle and his colleagues then kept the protein percent at 30 for the following 12 weeks and allowed subjects to eat as much as they felt they needed to satisfy hunger. Without being forced to maintain their previous 2400 calories (on average) per day, the study subjects immediately began to consume less. They continued eating less until the study ended. This resulted in an average weight loss of 5 kg (11.3 pounds). The authors noted that when the subjects ate less on a high protein diet, they did so by allowing fat percent, rather than carbohydrate, to decrease. Thus, they lost weight while maintaining carbohydrate intake, which suggests that *low-fat diets may simply work by increasing protein*. An important finding is that the higher protein diet did not produce weight loss when calories were maintained. The weight loss came only after the subjects were allowed to let the appetite suppressing effect of protein to alter their eating patterns. The laws of physics were not defied by the study, and calories still accounted for weight loss. While protein may change our metabolic rate or cause more energy to be used for digestion, in this study, those effects were not found, and the appetite suppressing effect and eating less were the not-so-mysterious cause of the weight loss.

Why would the body suppress appetite in the presence of increased protein? Doesn't the protein leverage framework propose that humans regulate diet to get maximum protein? Not exactly. The theory is that the body seeks an *optimum* amount of protein for health, reproduction, and longevity. Which brings us to the more critical concern of whether eating this way could actually harm human health. The weight losing aspect and appetite suppressing effects of high protein diets suggest that they work because the body is trying to protect itself from something harmful. Satiety from food could be seen as confirming that you've eaten the right thing, but early satiety, so much so that one naturally eats too few calories and loses weight, might suggest that the diet used for weight loss is actually unhealthy.

Simpson and Raubenheimer suggest that we can consider this question by examining other species. An entire chapter in *The Nature of Nutrition* is dedicated to possible mechanisms whereby species balance the risks and benefits of protein intake as they relate to growth, reproduction, and longevity. In a discussion of the concept of caloric restriction and longevity (the, perhaps kooky, notion that we can live longer by eating substantially less), they point out that restriction of protein is, in fact, the mediator of the life extending properties of calorie restricted diets. They report (with Lee and colleagues, *PNAS,* 2008) that fruit flies can live equal amounts of time on a wide variety of calories, but time of death is directly related to the ratio of protein to carbohydrate in the flies' diet. As they diluted the carbohydrate with more and more protein, the lifespan of the flies grew progressively shorter. There was a clear "dose-response" relationship between protein amount and risk of mortality, with risk growing in step-wise fashion with each increase in protein given. This has been shown to be true for crickets and rodents as well. Specific dietary manipulations suggest that it may be particular combinations of amino acids that act as the shorteners of life, with rat studies showing restricting methionine to be necessary for life extension. This implicates methionine as a potentially life shortening amino acid in these insect and animal models. While the pathways for a potential toxicity of protein are not known, there are corollary studies in humans that find higher amounts of protein showing negative health effects.

N. Santesso and colleagues published a review of dietary protein effects on health outcomes in the *European Journal of Clinical Nutrition* in 2012. They looked at over 100 studies of higher versus lower protein diets published in major journals to conclude that "higher protein diets probably improve adiposity, blood pressure and triglyceride levels, but these effects are small and need to be weighed against potential for harms." The harms examined in the study included more gastrointestinal symptoms and muscle cramping in high-protein groups, as well as some studies reporting increases in creatinine (a marker of kidney stress). The analysis was based on 3 month outcomes, so did not have anything to say about longevity.

In 2014, a paper by Morgan Levine and colleagues, caused a stir by suggesting that lower protein, not higher protein, was protective against several chronic diseases and risk of death. Looking at the NHANES database and assigning individuals to either a "low-protein" category of <10%, or "high protein" category of >20%, the authors showed that lower protein intake reduced risk of mortality from all causes, including cancer and diabetes. This was true only for the age group that was 50-65 years old. Those older than 65 had improvement in longevity with higher protein diets. Several experts expressed criticism of this study in interviews and social media, particularly objecting to the idea of categorizing diet by using only one dietary recall questionnaire and assuming that individuals do not change diet over decades of follow up. Nevertheless, the suggestion that there may be negative consequences of a higher protein diet need to be taken seriously.

The companies which fill our grocery store with the products we buy haven't heard of protein leverage. They aren't trying to design an optimal ecosystem from which we forage for superior nutrition. They are selling stuff. The Crunch Berry people are neither trying to hurt us nor help us. They just want to give us what we want at a price we will pay. Right now, we seem to be leaning toward protein. In fact, we are we are likely at the initial stage of a high protein experiment, much like the low-fat experiment of the 1980s and '90s. This took several years to ramp up and would take many more to ramp back down. We are very likely to see manifestations of this change at the group level.

The protein leverage hypothesis starts with the idea that the body has inherent wisdom which works to control food intake. It's possible that there will be no negative consequences of this consumer protein revolution, if our bodies naturally restore us to an optimum diet, in a better ecosystem, where protein is more readily available. Perhaps "protein water" is simply part of this needed re-balancing. But I think that's overly optimistic. Bodies seem to respond on a bell curve, so what works for a little needed weight loss for one person, or most, is bound to induce too much weight loss in a few. Just as the "fat is bad" notion was mis-applied to the general population, a "protein is good" mindset has the potential to cause harm to those who are already obtaining enough for optimum function. In a perspective article in the journal Obesity, Raubenheimer and colleagues suggest that the upper limits for protein set in the nutritional recommendations of various countries (USDA, AMDR, etc) may be as important as the lower limit. Balancing protein intake, not simply increasing it, is the key to optimizing health.

## How Is Protein Sensed and Balanced in the Body?

The body reacts to increasing protein in the diet with a counter-regulation that decreases appetite, apparently in an effort to avoid protein excess. But how is this accomplished? Somehow, the protein ingested, as it is broken down into its component amino acids, must be sensed, either by our individual cells or the brain. While the handling of the nitrogen contained in protein is thoroughly understood (the primary need for urination is to regulate nitrogen balance) sensing and controlling the concentration of the amino acids as they relate to our everyday need for repair and growth is more mysterious. The hypothalamus, which coordinates a variety of nerve inputs related to hunger and satiety, also functions to monitor the blood. Through this monitoring, the hypothalamus acts as a nutrient sensor for glucose, fatty acids and amino acids and uses this information in coordination with gut satiety signals to control our feeding.

But the protein leverage hypothesis proposes that there is a very direct link between protein intake and calories consumed, that somehow protein has a different, more powerful, effect on our metabolism than the other two macronutrients which are shown to fluctuate much more, without harming health. How does protein affect calorie consumption?

Recall (from Chapter 2) that calories cannot really be said to exist outside of the lab. We don't burn calories in the body, we burn fat, protein and carbohydrate after they've been digested and converted to energy. This energy takes the form of ATP within our body. So, we are not actually looking for a protein/calorie interaction, but rather a protein/ATP interaction. The question is: Can we find any mechanism which might link protein intake to ATP levels in our cells?

The difficulty with trying to study ATP is that the individual molecules exist only for moments within cells, as they are used perpetually to drive the chemical reactions that keep us alive, warm, repairing ourselves and growing. ATP can't be measured in the blood, urine, or spinal fluid. It'll be gone by the time you put a muscle biopsy under a microscope. For these reasons, we have always used "calories" and "joules" which denote heat energy as a stand-in for the energy we get from food. But this brings the limitation of not knowing how those lab measurements convert to our internal energy levels.

Recall that ATP stands for "adenosine *Tri* phosphate." This molecule gives up one of its charged phosphate groups to become ADP, or "adenosine *Di* phosphate," which quickly gets recharged to ATP or degrades further to AMP, "adenosine *Mono* phosphate." The three molecules keep their primary structure intact and vary only by whether they have one, two, or three phosphate groups attached. They perhaps can best be considered one molecule that exists in three energy states:

**AMP<—>ADP <—> ATP**

It is the giving and taking of the phosphate groups that drive the vast majority of chemical reactions that constitute animal life. When ATP levels are high, we can replicate our DNA, form enzymes, grow our cell structures, repair internal damage, move our muscles, digest our food, type on our computers . . . whatever it is we need to do. As ATP gets used up, AMP levels rise and it is important that the body sense this, in order to turn down all of the activities above, which are energy consuming.

If a scientist were to dream up a molecule which might serve as an indicator of energy levels within our cells, he would be hard-pressed to do better than AMPK. This molecule is part of a cascade of chemical reactions that are set in motion when AMP levels rise in a cell, which is why it is called "AMP *activated* kinase" or AMPK for short. AMPK then acts to conserve cellular energy by slowing DNA replication, protein creation, cell growth and division, heat production, etc. It serves as a regulator of the activity within each cell, so that when available energy is running low, the cell reduces its activities to preserve itself (this discussion based on Viollet 2010).

In addition to controlling cellular reactions, AMPK regulates the use of our two main fuel sources: fat and carbohydrate. Because the concentration of AMP is inversely related to the amount of glucose available, AMPK signals the cell to cease storing glucose as glycogen and to utilize fatty acids to replenish ATP supplies, instead of putting this excess energy into storage. It also encourages glycogen breakdown to counteract the decreasing glucose concentration in the cell.

The AMPK molecule is conserved through nearly all species down to single-celled yeast which have a very simple metabolism: When glucose is available, yeast grow and divide; when it is absent, they shut down to remain alive. AMPK is the means by which they accomplish this sensing. It does the same job, with some refinements, in our more complicated bodies. Human AMPK activity is also modulated by ATP directly (which inhibits it) so that it can be considered a direct stand-in for the AMP:ATP ratio at any given moment. This makes it an excellent candidate for a whole body energy sensor and indicator.

AMPK has a counterpart, called mTOR, which is more active when levels of ATP are high in the cell:

$$\uparrow \text{AMPK} \mathrel{<\!\!-} \text{AMP} \mathrel{<\!\!-\!\!>} \text{ADP} \mathrel{<\!\!-\!\!>} \text{ATP} \mathrel{-\!\!>} \uparrow \text{mTOR}$$

This molecule is the "mammalian Target of Rapamycin," which is a drug taken by transplant patients. That accident of naming doesn't help our discussion here. When we aren't talking about the medicine rapamycin, mTOR's normal every day role in the cell is to sense and communicate that ATP levels are rising. mTOR turns on processes which require a lot of energy, such as copying DNA, encouraging cell growth and reproduction, reinforcing cellular structure, creating enzymes necessary for chemical reactions, storing excess glucose as glycogen, and generating heat along the way. In the same way that AMPK gets to work when AMP signals low energy, mTOR ramps up when ATP signals that energy is abundant. AMPK is the "hunker down and wait" signal; mTOR is the "times are good" signal. AMPK and mTOR are also able to interact with each other directly, with AMPK acting to inhibit mTOR activity in order to shut down energy wasting processes more quickly.

With regard to uncovering the mechanisms of protein leverage, it has been shown that amino acids directly affect the activity levels of both AMPK and mTOR. The amino acid leucine seems to exert the strongest signal to the cells that protein is present. The body seems to put this in the "times are good" category. Leucine acts to turn off the actions of AMPK and turn on the actions of mTOR. This correlates well with the observation that protein is satiating: mTOR acts when nutrients are available and AMPK when they are absent.

Because amino acids seem to have this ability, which is not observed with carbohydrate or fat, the possibility presents itself that amino acids acting on the AMPK and mTOR system may be how protein exerts more influence on our eating behavior than those other nutrients. The body does not stop eating until it has what it wants. The protein leverage hypothesis contends that protein is what it wants most. When enough protein is present, the signal that the cells are in good energy standing seems to run through mTOR and AMPK.

Since both AMPK and mTOR pathways are carried out within cells and neither molecule travels through the body in the circulation, it would seem that neither could be considered a *whole body* energy sensor. However, these very same pathways are active in the hypothalamus, which governs our energy regulation. In addition to receiving signals of nutrient status from the gut via the nervous system, the cells of the hypothalamus, through their interaction with the blood, are subject to the same regulation by protein's availability as every other cell in the body. In the presence of increased amino acids, the hypothalamus will have decreased AMPK activity and increased mTOR activity, reflecting a nutrient replete status. These alterations in activity have been shown to act as a satiety signal to the hypothalamus which is responsible for the deciding whether or not we eat. The AMPK and mTOR activity levels in the hypothalamus may be the key to understanding why protein satisfies hunger and why the protein leverage effect occurs.

Because so much of our attention, when it comes to nutrition questions, is focused on the problem of obesity, any new possible solution is bound to be greeted with enthusiasm by the public. It is quite possible that increasing protein in the food supply in response to consumer demand will act to slow or even reverse obesity rates. Protein bars and shakes are everywhere you look now and it seems that "high protein" is the new "low-carb" or "low-fat." However, the pathways we have just brought into the discussion can serve to highlight how intricately balanced are the factors related to energy consumption and our overall health. If protein consumption decreases appetite by significantly altering the activity of such ubiquitous molecules as AMPK and mTOR, it is highly unlikely that it could do this without having unexpected consequences.

I have always counseled patients that, in my opinion, weight loss medications don't seem to work, and if one was ever to work well, you wouldn't want to take it, because it could only do so by disrupting many body systems at once, causing problems perhaps worse than obesity. The possibility that the same could be true for systematically increasing protein consumption needs to be examined before we celebrate the changes we are seeing in the food supply.

## References:

Weigle, DS, et. al. A high-protein diet induces sustained reductions in appetite, ad libitum caloric intake, and body weight despite compensatory changes in diurnal plasma leptin and ghrelin concentrations. *American Journal of Clinical Nutrition* 2005, 82(1): 41-48.

Lee, KP, et. al. Lifespan and reproduction in Drosophilia: New insights from nutritional geometry. *PNAS* 2008, 105: 2498-2503.

Simpson, SJ, Le Couteur, DG, Rabenheimer, D. Putting the balance back in Diet. *Cell* 2015, 161(1): 18-23.

Santesso, N, et. al. Effects of higher versus lower protein diets on health outcomes: a systematic review and meta-analysis. *European Journal of Clinical Nutrition* 2012, 66(7): 780-788.

Levine, ME, et. al. Low-protein intake is associated with a major reduction in IGF-1, cancer and overall mortality in the 65 and younger but not older population. *Cell Metabolism* 2014, 19(3): 407-417.

Raubenheimer, et. al. Integrating Nutrients, Foods, Diets, and Appetites with Obesity and Cardiometabolic Health. *Obesity* 2015, 23(9): 1741-42.

Viollet B. et. al. AMPK inhibition in health and disease. *Critical Reviews In Biochemistry And Molecular Biology* 2010, 45(4): 276-295.

# Chapter 8

## You Can't Run It Off

Picture this: An anxious patient sits in the doctor's exam room. He has handed his health questionnaire to the receptionist detailing his diabetes, cholesterol problems, and hypertension. The nurse has checked his height and weight and recorded the numbers in his chart. He is ready for advice from the obesity doctor, hoping to learn how to get rid of the 100 pounds that have crept onto his body over the last few decades. The doctor enters and says, "Wow, Mr. Jones, that's quite an exercise problem you have there! How long have you been suffering from this exercise condition?"

*That would be a strange beginning, wouldn't it?*

We know, intuitively, that obesity and the metabolic diseases are primarily food-related and any weight loss patient would first and foremost expect that it would be diet that needs to be addressed by the obesity specialist. But, like anyone inexperienced in treating obesity, I initially made the assumption that to help people lose weight, you would need to address *both* diet and exercise. When my first clinic opened in 2011, I asked the hospital for three staff members: a dietitian, a health coach and a fitness trainer. We were slow to find the right trainer and a couple months after opening, I had them cancel the job posting.

In the first several weeks, I discovered that weight loss, for the very heavy patients I was seeing (I was the medical doctor in a bariatric surgery office, so all the patients were at least 100 pounds over "ideal" weight) had little to do with activity. Successful patients appeared to be those who made big changes in diet. I found that my patients who simultaneously took it upon themselves to exercise (I was not recommending it) did no better than those that didn't. In fact, they seemed to be having a tougher time, perhaps by wasting too much effort on the wrong part of the energy balance equation.

Then, there were all the issues with injuries. Not surprisingly, when one is a very heavy middle-aged person who suddenly begins an aggressive exercise program, injuries are common. One afternoon, I got frustrated and left a somewhat cryptic message for Lance Farrell, the owner of a local chain of martial arts-based fitness centers:

"Please stop breaking my patients' feet."

Lance is a positive, confident guy, so instead of getting defensive, he got in touch with our office to set up a meeting to discuss what was going on. I explained that I had met three patients in three months who had recently dropped out of his fitness challenge course because rising up on one foot to perform martial arts kicks had caused stress fractures in the metatarsal bones of their feet. "Like a dancer's fracture?" Lance asked, and I knew I'd found an intelligent collaborator.

Working together over the following few months, we designed an alternative program to his "boot camp" style competition. This involved screening heavier and sicker individuals more carefully and offering a run-in program to get them ready for the full-on daily intensity of the "extreme bodyshaping" course that the gyms are famous for. It worked well, prevented injuries, provided an outreach to people who otherwise would eschew work-out programs and continues to run in the Des Moines facilities. For Lance, it worked out perfectly. For me, the entire episode made me question how important exercise really should be for people who are not naturally athletic.

The idea that we should exercise to help with weight loss is logical enough. Our body weight is the cumulative result of a daily energy balance between what we put in and what we use. Since exercise uses energy, it would seem reasonable to increase the "out" side of the equation while simultaneously reducing what goes "in." But how big of an impact can exercise have? Recall the breakdown of energy expenditure:

$$E = DIT + PA + RMR + NEAT$$

Where "E" has its four components (as discussed in Chapter 2): diet induced thermogenesis (DIT), which is the amount of energy we use digesting our food, plus physical activity (PA) like running and working out, resting metabolic rate (RMR, what's needed to keep the organs working), and "non-exercise activity thermogenesis," which we call NEAT (including fidgeting, posture maintenance and all other movements not measurable as PA).

These factors vary between individuals, but the average percentage of calories burned by each of the factors is generally agreed to be roughly:

—RMR: 60-65%

—DIT: 5-10%

—PA: 20%

—NEAT: 10%

(Extrapolated from Thomas, 2009)

These factors vary depending upon age, weight, activity level, etc. But no matter what, the vast majority of our energy is spent simply keeping the organs functioning and digesting our food. The brain alone accounts for 18% of energy burned daily, more than you can spend in deliberate exercise. At first glance, one might be tempted to think that increasing "PA" by exercising, would, over time, make the difference between lean and obese. But one needs to consider that physical activity includes *all* of your activity while awake, 16 hours or more of movement, not just your exercise. This includes getting ready for work, dressing, showering, walking to and fro, etc. From a strictly mathematical standpoint, even if you chose to exercise an hour a day, every day (and very few of us can keep up a commitment like that) *you would be acting on only 1/16th of 20% of your metabolism.* Everyone who exercises an hour a day, spends 23 hours per day not exercising. There is simply no way around this.

This is borne out in studies which assess the effect of formal exercise on weight. In a 2005 review in the *International Journal of Obesity,* Curioni and Lorenco examined the results of studies which compared diet alone with a diet + exercise prescription, (choosing only studies which accurately measured both parameters). They found, when synthesizing the results of the six trials that met their rigid criteria for quality, that exercise led to a (statistically insignificant) greater weight loss of 6.5 pounds in the short term and a 4 pound greater (again insignificant statistically) weight loss at one year. This was on top of a one year average weight loss of 10 pounds across all studies.

In a more recent review published in the *American Journal of Medicine*, researchers looked at the impact of aerobic exercise without dietary changes, on 3 month and 12 month outcomes (Thorogood, 2011). Fourteen randomized controlled trials were analyzed to show that aerobic exercise of 120 minutes per week produced very modest weight losses of 2-4 pounds at 3 months which were maintained at the end of a year. There were also small improvements in waist circumference (one inch) and blood pressure (2 mmHg).

As I've pointed out previously regarding weight loss results, we could delve deeper into these studies, try to assess whether resistance routines are better than aerobic exercise, or interval training beats them both, but what's the point? The details don't matter much when the big picture analysis gives results of 2-6 pounds! Obesity is a complex medical disorder with identifiable hormonal, metabolic, neurologic derangements in the context of large amounts of weight gain. If exercising consistently for a year is only going to improve weight by single digits, we need not impose this extra burden on our patients, or ourselves.

Many physicians argue that the advice to increase exercise is not really about pounds on the scale, but measurable risks for disease. Exercise improves cholesterol, blood pressure and inflammation, even without much weight loss. Leaving aside for the moment the fact that patients themselves do, in fact, measure success in terms of pounds, not mmHg blood pressure or mg/dL cholesterol, what amount of exercise would be required to change medical risk?

This question was addressed by Cris Slentz and colleagues in "Exercise, Abdominal Obesity and Metabolic Risk: Evidence for a Dose Response." In this 2009 paper, the researchers looked at how much and how hard we need exercise to improve our risk for diabetes and heart disease. They took volunteers and broke them into three groups: The first was advised to exercise at low amount/moderate intensity (equivalent to walking 12 miles per week). The second was asked to exercise at low amount/vigorous intensity (jogging 12 miles per week). The third was set to high amount at vigorous intensity (jogging 20 miles per week —75% VO2max). With these three groups they assessed the effect of the different programs on the participants' risk factors for metabolic disease over the course of six months.

Their findings were a mix of good and bad news. The good news was, participants were able control their diabetes and heart disease risk by exercise. The bad news was, it took a lot of exercise to achieve meaningful results. Dr. Slentz and colleagues measured the LDL particle number, LDL particle size and the HDL size in

158

the subjects. They also looked at visceral fat (waist circumference) and the amount of exercise needed just to lose some weight. They then plotted the improvement in these numbers against a baseline sedentary group to calculate how much exercise it takes to "break even." They asked: How much do people need to exercise before they begin to achieve a meaningful improvement in each of these parameters?

### *Miles per week needed before improvement begins:*

—Fat mass: 4

—LDL size: 7

—Lose weight: 8

—HDL: 10

—Visceral fat: 13

—LDL #: 13

These were the minimum amounts needed to see *any effect at all.* In other words: A person could walk seven extra miles per week and see no change in weight. After this "break-even" number, the improvement curves rose fairly swiftly in the positive direction with a general "more is better" relationship to the number of miles. What they found when they looked specifically at the measures most closely related to diabetes (triglycerides, insulin resistance, and a metabolic score) was that walking seemed to improve those factors more than running.

The amount of exercise a person considers "a lot," is, of course, relative. Perhaps 13 miles sounds like a minimal weekly amount of walking or jogging to some, but I would counter that would only be to someone who isn't obese and doesn't work with very obese patients. If I had recommended 2 miles a day as the minimum dose of exercise to get measurable risk reduction to my patients, a good deal would have answered that if they could walk two miles a day, they wouldn't need to come see me at all! And I would have agreed.

So exercise doesn't easily translate to weight loss in individuals. But surely if you get large groups of people to increase exercise, you can detect an improvement in population health over time. *Right?*

This hypothesis was examined in an analysis that was published by Ali Mokdad's group in 2013, which showed that increasing physical activity rates on a county by county basis did not have a beneficial effect on obesity rates. They took survey data from the Behavioral Risk Factor Surveillance System (BRFSS) and the National Health and Nutrition Examination Survey (NHANES) to assess how well activity patterns correlate with obesity patterns by county, comparing changes over 10 years.

What they found was that there is almost no correlation between rising activity levels in particular counties and improvements in obesity rates in those counties. They concluded that "for every 1 percentage point increase in physical activity prevalence, obesity prevalence was 0.11 percentage points lower." Unfortunately, they don't explain, "lower than what," but by reading the paper several times I deciphered that they meant "lower than the rise in obesity that would have been expected." So they are talking about a very slight *decrease* in the rate of *increase* in obesity, for those counties that saw more physical activity over ten years. As they reported a 10:1 ratio cause to effect, it is safe to say that the study showed essentially no value, in terms of county-level obesity rates, attributable to increasing activity levels in any county over a ten year period.

The researchers didn't say that counties with more exercisers didn't have a lower baseline obesity rate (they generally do), but simply that the cause and effect you might wish for if you were applying for a grant (like, that your plans to build bicycle paths will reduce the county obesity rate) is hard to find in the data. We don't know if all those people in Douglas County, Colorado (which had the lowest obesity rates and highest exercise rates) are skinny because they hike and bike so much or whether all the skinny people that live there happened to be hikers and bikers who moved to Colorado to do that stuff. We don't know anything about the reasons behind the baseline correlations. What we do know is that the counties that saw the biggest increase in activity over a decade did not become skinny and those that decreased activity did not become heavier than expected.

These results were worth publishing and I bring them into the discussion here because they are surprising: The proposition that we should exercise more to decrease obesity rates seems like it would be so clear that you are almost testing a tautology. This comes from our conflating fitness with weight loss. We use obesity as the inspiration for bike paths and trail building and public health campaigns to get people outside, assuming that exercise *has to be* a good thing. However, it has little to do with weight one way or another: not on an individual level, not on a county level and not on a national level. If we decide that exercise is something universally good and want to promote it, then it needs to be for its own sake, not as a response to the obesity epidemic.

## If Exercise Doesn't Work, How About Activity?

From the discussion the above, we can reject the notion that weight loss can be bought with a gym membership. But before we go dismissing the calorie burning side of the energy equation altogether, we should consider an aspect of movement that actually does have real merit and some good scientific reinforcement.

I have noticed, on many occasions, while taking a patient's weight history, that jobs seem to make a difference. It is common for people to tell me that they lost 30 pounds after taking a job in construction, or that they gained 30 pounds when they got promoted to supervisor and had to sit at a desk all day. Truck drivers have inordinately high rates of obesity, with good reason: They are literally paid to sit still.

This type of change is not dealing with "exercise" but with all-day measures of physical activity and "NEAT." James Levine, a doctor at the Mayo Clinic has done more to popularize the idea that daily movement is important for weight control than any other researcher. While he didn't "discover" the concept of "non-exercise activity thermogenesis," he has led the research to characterize it and popularized it as a concept.

He laid out his ideas in a 2004 paper in the *American Journal of Physiology*. In this discussion, Dr. Levine shows that the basal metabolism (RMR in the equation) and the DIT (energy for digesting food) fluctuate very little. But the NEAT can be as little as 15% in a sedentary person and up to 50% of total energy expenditure in a very active person. Dr. Levine argues that "for the vast majority of dwellers in developed countries, exercise-related activity thermogenesis is negligible or zero." Thus, all "PA" can be subsumed into the term "NEAT." He then compares the energy lost to various activities which aren't required due to modernization and labor saving devices. He proposes a philosophically pleasing idea: Modern life has made us heavy by making things too easy.

If life is too easy in our modern environment, then the solution would be to find ways to make it harder again. Levine published his sentiments on this subject in a 2009 book entitled *Move a Little, Lose a Lot*. In it, he makes a very forceful and compelling argument that our approach to general, everyday living, rather than our approach to formal exercise, can make a difference for weight. He relates the story of how he personally realized the importance of NEAT by analyzing the movements of naturally lean and naturally obese subjects. The lean individuals burned 300+ calories more per day in incidental movements, mostly standing and walking. He then argues that this is enough to account for the differences found in individuals' responses to weight loss interventions.

It's hard to argue with the few data points he presents. But his conclusions: that we should incorporate standing work stations, take our meetings walking and even read his book while pacing (he recommends this), seem a bit bizarre to me. He describes his lab as a hive of restless activity, where everyone stands, walks and fidgets through all productive activity, presumably when they are not annoying their co-workers by jiggling on an exercise ball in lieu of a chair. He suggests a treadmill in front of the TV at home and has designed a treadmill desk. I wonder if the Mayo Clinic NEAT laboratory is largely filled with the already fit and the "used to be fit, but just need to get back into it" crowd that is common in medical academia. His book does document occasional examples of heavier patients seeing real improvements in health parameters. But the majority of the case study examples involve people losing 10 or 15 pounds and "feeling great." I suspect he is largely preaching to the converted and that few truly obese patients will get much from his recommendations.

The medical literature supports that we are all wired differently with regard to activity. In a recently published trial in the journal *Obesity* (Herrmann, 2015), researchers assigned a group of 74 overweight and obese adults to a five day per week exercise regimen for 10 months. The outcomes, as in most studies, were variable, in terms of amount of weight lost from the program. To further describe this natural variability, the researchers divided the participants into "responders" and "non-responders" to the intervention by whether they lost more than 5% of body weight. They showed that responders were able to eat less, burn more energy between sessions, and also increase non-exercise activity. The "non-responders" (about half of the group) were the people whose natural response was to decrease activity between sessions, naturally slow metabolism and eat a bit more to make up for the exercise. This argues that whether we are going to feel great and get fit with an instruction to move more may not be something we can choose.

Many of my patients seemed to grasp this intuitively when we discussed their past history. When a new exercise idea was proposed by a patient, I would usually respond with "Well, did you used to work out a lot, when you were lighter?" If the answer was "No," I would generally recommend against relying on exercise. If the answer was "Yes, I used to be a jock," then I generally supported starting back into it. It seemed very likely to me that grade school gym class had already sorted out personal talents and predilections with regard to athletics. With regard to the "move more" hypothesis of Dr. Levine, I would agree that trying to increase all-day activity makes more sense than trying to burn calories for an hour in the gym. But I am not convinced that it is the difference between the heavy and the lean. I think it's more likely the difference between the lean and the *leaner*.

Not everyone is an athlete. That's okay. But when I try to gently move the conversation with patients away from exercise and toward food issues, I always sense some disappointment. The fact is that losing weight is about "getting healthy" for most patients. Even knowing that exercise can't burn enough calories to matter, most people want to include exercise in a weight loss effort because the drive for thinness is an attempt to feel better. People assume that those who exercise feel better than those who don't. I can't argue with that logic.

In my practice, after years of internally debating what's best, I settled on a simple counseling pattern that worked for most of my patients: exercise if it makes you feel good, don't exercise if it makes you feel bad, or if you can't get into a groove. Focus on increasing walking distance over time with the goal of eventually being able to walk as much as you want without your weight limiting you. Be aware that your approach has to work in sickness and in health, which includes orthopedic injuries that can keep you out of the gym for months. Just like with diet, try to utilize ideas that are possible to maintain for the long term, hopefully a lifetime.

## References:

Slentz, C. et. al. Exercise, abdominal obesity, skeletal muscle and metabolic risk: evidence for a dose response. *Obesity* 2009, 17 (supp3).

Dwyer-Lindgren, L. et. al. Prevalence of physical activity and obesity in US counties, 2001-2011: a road map for action. *Population Health Metrics* 2013, 11(7).

Thomas, DM. et al. A mathematical model of weight change with adaptation. *Math, Biosciences and Engineering* 2009, 6(4): 873-887.

Curioni, CC. Lourenco, PM. Long-term weight loss after diet and exercise: a systematic review. *International Journal of Obesity* 2005, 29(10): 1168-1174.

Thorogood A. et. al. Isolated aerobic exercise and weight loss: a systematic review and meta-analysis of randomized controlled trials. *American Journal of Medicine* 2011, 124 (8): 747-755.

Levine, JA. Nonexercise activity thermogenesis (NEAT): environment and biology. *American Journal of Physiology - Endocrinology and Metabolism* 2004, 286(5): E675-E685.

Levine, JA. *Move a Little, Lose a Lot*. New York: Crown Publishing, 2009.

Herrmann SD. et. al. Energy intake, nonexercise physical activity, and weight loss in responders and nonresponders: The Midwest Exercise Trial 2. *Obesity* 2015, 23(8): 1539-1549.

# Chapter 9

## Are All Weight Loss Doctors Quacks?

Ben Goldacre, whom I hold in high esteem, has repeatedly contended that anyone espousing diet philosophies to others is practicing quackery. Eating, he argues, does not require scientific scrutiny, nor does it take any specialized knowledge to get healthier: Walk a little, ride a bike, eat your veggies . . . who needs a doctor to tell them to do those things? In fact, on his website, he sells T-shirts with a picture of a large rubber ducky and underneath the caption is simply, "Nutritionist."

Dr. Goldacre is a British physician who rails against quacks and charlatans. His book, *Bad Science,* is a funny, insightful, merciless critique of lazy and dishonest scientists. I think he's on the right side of almost every argument he's engaged in (and he's engaged in several at most times). So it troubles me that he might consider what I did in practice and the science that I write about currently, as quackery.

While practicing "obesity medicine" for four years, I often contemplated what the doctor's role in nutrition counseling should be. I am always a little perturbed by the label of "nutritionist," because I don't really know what the term means. There are dietitians, physicians, counselors —but what exactly is a nutritionist? We use the term here too (so it's not just a British-U.S. translation problem), but I've never met one. From reading Goldacre's blog and watching some of his interviews, it seems that he's mostly concerned about those who peddle weight loss solutions using pseudoscience and even fake degrees from non-existent institutions. So maybe I'm safe —I'm not doing those things. But he goes on to state things of this nature, often:

*"And the grandiose nutritionism-peddling columnists from Sunday magazines, even if they do recommend you eat some particular nut because it contains lots of vitamin G and selenium, are still basically recommending fruit and veg. Everyone knows basic dietary advice, and they don't need a nutritionist, doctor, alternative therapist or journalist, to tell them. They need their mum."* —Bad Science blog post 6/2/05.

So the question, for a doc like me, is whether the whole idea of practicing "obesity medicine," even when we aren't advocating for our favorite vitamin or magic ingredient, is legitimate; or is it all just quackery?

Let's begin to answer this quackery charge by observing that, in the U.S. at least, there is no legitimate obesity specialization on a residency or fellowship level. This is not to say that there won't be soon. The board of medical specialties didn't recognize Family Practice until the 1970s; so these things do change as practice models change. But, currently, you could not choose to be an obesity doctor (bariatrician) coming straight out of medical school. To become an obesity doctor, you currently need to do a full residency of some sort, then go find extra training. This is to say, you are not practicing in a recognized, accredited field when you say you practice bariatrics, obesity medicine, or (cringe) weight loss.

There are two major societies that support continuing education conferences which help U.S. physicians learn some obesity science. I've been a member of both at different times. The American Society of Bariatric Physicians (ASBP) is mostly geared toward helping primary care doctors improve their treatment of obesity-related conditions, and it helps them determine how to offer "weight loss," to existing patients.

At ASBP conferences, one can learn the basic science that underpins weight regulation: some endocrinology, some nutrition, some neurology and some behavior. Indications for when to use medications and when to consult bariatric surgeons are taught. The society promotes best practices, advocates against dangerous or silly treatments (like HCG) through position papers, creates free downloadable algorithms, etc. Successful weight loss doctors and researchers active in the field are members and run the meetings. They orient you to history, including the history of mistakes like Fen-Phen "pill-mills" and teach one how not to fall into becoming the "wrong sort" of weight loss doctor. This is the more practical of the two societies. This is where you learn "how to do it."

The second society is dubbed simply "The Obesity Society." It is heavily skewed toward research and the yearly conference is a bit closer to what you'd experience at the scientific conferences of any specialty: You would be bored out of your mind unless this was your passion. The Obesity Society is the parent organization running the journal *Obesity* which contains the same legitimate science you'd find in any peer-reviewed journal. This is not to suggest that ASBP is not scientific, but TOS is more research-oriented and ASBP more practice-oriented.

Both of these societies are now offering "board certification," by testing through a central authority called the American Board of Obesity Medicine. This is not the same as being board certified in one's specialty, which denotes that a physician has done between one and six full-time years of extra work after internship. These certifications are tests that one can take after a moderate number of hours accumulated at conferences, along with some mentoring.

How patients are supposed to know that physicians promoting themselves as "board certified" from these societies is not equivalent to the way the term is used for something like "board certified neurosurgeon," I'm not sure. The term borders on misleading, in my opinion. A "certificate of additional training" from the "society" rather than "certification" from a "board" would more accurately reflect what the doctor has gone through.

That being said, the two societies point out that this is how new specialties become recognized: bringing together scientists and practitioners with common interests, educating new members, increasing research funding, setting practice standards . . . until teaching hospitals begin to create fellowships and full residencies. Obesity medicine is likely in this transition.

But is what is taught and practiced quackery, in the Ben Goldacre sense? I would answer with a definitive *No*. The science is certainly not quackery. It's about digestion, metabolic pathways, neuro-endocrine signaling, exactly as one might expect. However, we run into some problems when we try to figure out how one is supposed to put any of this scientific knowledge into practice.

Contrary to what some might think, becoming a weight loss physician is not an easy path to riches. Since there is essentially no insurance reimbursement in the U.S. for this activity, one is either forced to bill weight management as lifestyle counseling (for $15 per half hour visit) or bill under whichever disease a patient has that is co-morbid, such as diabetes. But one doesn't get any "extra" reimbursement for choosing to treat diabetes with a diet program in addition to writing a quick prescription. Because it is so difficult to get reimbursed for anything *other than* writing a prescription, the ASBP does run a two day conference helping doctors get started on the business of running a clinic based on behavior modification: motivational interviewing, journaling one's food, and exercise prescription. The "business" teaching can feel a little . . . bourgeois. . . . or maybe gauche (I don't know why there isn't a word in English for this) for physicians, who generally aren't comfortable considering medicine a business.

Because payment from insurance is essentially non-existent, there are certainly are some physicians who decide to chuck the whole idea of traditional billing and run a "cash only" weight loss clinic. We have several words for this in English and I will let the reader choose one mentally as I point out that the way that one gets paid does not, in and of itself, mean that the physician is practicing quackery. You can't run a business without being paid and so far, insurance essentially does not pay U.S. doctors for this work.

To be a quack, one has to hold scientifically unsubstantiated views and to espouse them to less educated consumers of health care, generally for self-gain. I haven't run into this in the medical colleagues I've met at these meetings. The practitioners and researchers at society conferences are just professionals who see a need, care about people's health and think that this condition deserves more attention. They see what obesity does to the health of their patients and they want to help through educating themselves on how the condition arises and what are the best treatments . . . just as they would for any other condition.

Sure, there are always oddballs in a large society. There can be the occasional lecture with a contrarian view that goes against established science, such as contending that many more people need testosterone treatment, or Vitamin D, or thyroid hormone, than are currently getting it. In the past, I've attended some talks that could rightfully be categorized as "disease mongering" as well, with suggested changes of thresholds for obesity definition, or certain nutrition deficiency states. But I've never been to a conference for any discipline where every presentation matches my pre-conceived notions about best diagnoses and treatment. Fortunately, the oddball factor and disease mongering is rare in obesity science education. Most importantly, the societies promoting that we take the condition of obesity more seriously wish to apply the same scientific rigor to studying weight problems as we do for everything else. They are what will lead us *away* from disease mongering and quackery, not toward it.

The more immediate question, for the consumer, or to a colleague considering a referral, is whether *this* weight loss doctor is a quack.

***Warning signs might include:***

*—Selling products for cash in clinic*

*—Advertising a "program" that runs for a period of time*

*—Storefront location, rather than traditional clinic location*

*—A single answer for all cases of obesity (low-carb or get out!)*

*—Heavy use of medications off-label*

*—Use of "alternative" weight loss treatments like teas and supplements*

*—Excessive advertisement*

*—All patients are given a standard expensive battery of lab tests, regardless of whether their record already has tested sugar, thyroid, lipids, etc. Or, unusual tests are run to look for trace nutritional deficiencies*

There are, of course, exceptions to all of these. In large cities, storefront locations might be what's available. Providing some supplements to counteract a very low-calorie diet program might not be mercenary, etc. Everything in its place. But you should get the feeling that your "weight loss doctor" is actually acting like a doctor. It should feel like a regular clinic, not a vitamin shop. This is mostly a list of things that show the doctor is putting a commercial interest ahead of good medical practice. It doesn't guarantee quackery. But where there is too much commercial interest, the patient's health is likely at risk.

### *Signs that your weight loss doctor is practicing legitimately:*

*—You have a normal office visit in a clinic*

*—You have a medical history taken*

*—You are examined —like, the stethoscope part, not just height, weight and skin pinching*

*—Treatment advice takes into account your age, goals, medical problems, history, medications*

*—You are engaged in shared decision making which includes not trying things that have failed you in the past (low-carb or get out!)*

*—Medications should be optional and adjunctive to treatment. You should not be showing up once a month to get your "diet pill" prescription*

### *Things that would reassure me:*

*—My own doctor referred me*

*—The doctor has privileges at the local hospital*

*—He/She can account for his/her interest in obesity as a medical problem*

*—The doctor has an interest in the diseases that parallel obesity: heart disease, PCOS, infertility, type 2 diabetes, lipid problems. If your doctor is only interested in pounds on the scale, do you really need a doctor?*

*—Membership in either the American Society of Bariatric Physisians or The Obesity Society*

Another way to know if you've come to the office of someone with an actual interest in the condition of obesity is by looking around the waiting room. Do you see big people there? Are there people in wheelchairs? Sick people, like a normal doctor's office? Real doctors enjoy the challenge of sick patients and there should be signs that your obesity doctor is actually helping those who need it most.

Getting back to this issue of whether you need a doctor or a "mum" to address obesity . . . I'm going to just cut Ben Goldacre some slack and assume that he is not purposely trying to denigrate people or deny that there is real pain associated with severe obesity. I know he understands that there is a tremendous wealth of hormonal and neurological complexity underpinning food intake, appetite, energy regulation, and digestion. There can't really be a debate about whether metabolism is a legitimate scientific subject of inquiry: It's using the same biology, physiology, and pathophysiology as all the other fields we physicians spend our time worrying about. I'm going to assume that it's not *obesity* that he thinks we should talk to "Mum" about, but weight loss —Or even more specifically, "how one should eat."

## Does Obesity Need Its Own Specialty?

Do we need to go to a doctor to find out what and how much to eat? Should the doctors who become knowledgeable regarding mechanisms of adipose tissue regulation and energy balance spend their clinical time doing weight loss counseling? Probably not. I personally happened to be fairly good at counseling people how to eat, when I did it, but that part of the job is not really medical practice. Medical practice should consist of diagnosing and treating illness. I was educating, coaching, coaxing, cajoling, commiserating . . . but not really acting as a physician.

Does this mean that doctors should leave all questions regarding obesity to Weight Watchers and other commercial problems, since much of it is not medical? Absolutely not. We need doctors to take an interest in this science to help people avoid wasted time and dangerous programs. We need doctors educated enough in what actually works safely that they can persuade patients, using rational scientific explanations, against silly liquid diets, detox regimens, fasts, highly restrictive programs —all the fad nonsense. And we can't do this if we haven't actually studied any of it. Ideally, a physician should know enough to direct a team that includes a dietitian and a health coach, but the physician should not get confused (as I often did) and begin to actually *do* those jobs.

When I see how The Obesity Society and the ASBP have grown in the decade I've been attending their conferences, I have little doubt that we are effectively building a new specialty around this condition. It is specialized knowledge that gets taught. When I discuss anything about obesity in any detail with another physician, it is clear that the field contains its own terms and knowledge that are not part of general medical training. Like any field, there are jargon and minutia that don't translate directly to patient care and aren't necessary for every doctor to know. There needs to be a group of practitioners utilizing the new knowledge.

As the basic science knowledge base grows regarding obesity, we are getting a very clear picture of pathways that control normal regulation and what goes wrong with these biological processes as people becomes obese. This is how the scientific method informs medical practice. It's not the science of how to remember to eat your fruits and veggies that the researchers are examining. Nor is it quack theories about trace minerals and anti-oxidants from pomegranates. It's cell biology, biochemistry and pathophysiology they are elucidating and helping interested physicians to understand.

That being said, I don't see why we need to create a new specialty around this particular condition any more than we create a specialty solely around diabetes, high cholesterol or hypertension. Obesity fits just fine within known medical science and there is one specialty that is perfectly situated to take control of its management. It seems to me that the discipline of endocrinology, which does much of the serious clinical research in obesity, should be well-positioned to take leadership of the medical approach to this problem. Couldn't metabolism problems related to obesity (not just diabetes) become a sub-discipline within their field? Could they not include obesity medicine as an integral part of their education and ongoing training after residency? How about a two-year medical bariatric fellowship for endocrinologists after they are done getting trained in rare stuff they will rarely see in their day-to-day practice?

Currently, if you go to an endocrinologist to be worked up for excessive weight gain, he will make sure your thyroid is normal, your adrenals and pituitary don't have tumors, then send you back to your primary doc with reassurance that you *don't have an endocrine problem*. What type of problem is excessive growth of a certain body tissue type due to internal regulation abnormalities, if not an endocrine one? Granted, there are some endocrinologists involved in important ways in the societies I've discussed above (in some cases running things), but why are we training a whole new population of quasi-endocrinologists in the pathways of energy regulation and how the brain responds to bodily needs, when the endocrine docs already know this stuff better than we ever could? Perhaps the endocrinologists feel that weight loss is too unimportant of a subject to occupy their time. Perhaps there is still a general lack of appreciation of central regulation of obesity by hormones, in cases where that regulation is altered by food rather than a tumor. But, we need to be clear: Some people are 200 pounds overweight. Whether their adrenals and thyroid levels are normal or not, they need doctors who understand what's different about them. We need doctors to generally recognize and be able to handle the things that go wrong in the bodies of our heaviest patients. We *do not* need doctors pushing products and promises.

With regard to these questions, I always tried to keep a critical watch on my own practice, avoiding one-size-fits-all solutions and prescribing weight loss medications only rarely (I didn't find them very helpful). After I'd been working in obesity medicine for about a year, an opportunity presented itself to provide a meal replacement program to patients. It smacked of commercialism and I was reluctant at first. But wanting to be scientific about it, I saw no reason to dismiss it without trial. We brought in the program for a test run and some patients did very well. I began to compare the results of the meal replacement program to my standard advice and realized that, with all the meal replacement patients eating a standardized diet, we could test some questions about calories.

In 2013, I reached out to Kevin Hall at the NIH with a proposition for a research paper. We looked at a database of my clients participating in the supervised medical weight loss program with meal replacement. This program is terribly strict, supplying most of the food to the clients and asking only that they supplement with two cups of fresh vegetables and a "real" protein source of chicken, lean beef, or fish for dinner. Strict adherence to the diet provides between 900 and 1100 calories. It's a low-carb, low-fat, low-calorie diet, that is, by design, also a higher protein diet . . . since you cut everything else.

Whether the clients are adhering to this type of meal replacement diet is pretty simple: If they lose a ton of weight, they are adherent. The plan provides far too few calories for pretty much everyone, so if your patient comes in having stayed the same for more than a week, you can be pretty sure there has been some deviation from the program. We reviewed records from over 100 patients and found 49 for whom compliance seemed very tight for at least four weeks (based on the clinic notes which documented the patients' self-assessment on adherence). Then we asked: If one is extremely compliant to a rigid diet program, does the weight loss match what a mathematical model would predict?

The reason this is even in doubt is that pretty much every mathematical model will over-estimate the weight loss seen in a real, outpatient, free-living subject. Kevin and I wondered if that was due to some inherent flaw in these models, or whether free-living people are simply never compliant with recommendations (actually Kevin probably didn't wonder at all, because he's a scientist; but I'm just a clinician, so I truly wondered if there was some mysterious explanation of variable weight loss outcomes). With this very strict regimen and the close follow up, we were able to see how the weight loss of truly compliant patients added up. We plugged patients' height, weight, age, sex, and activity level into the NIH body weight simulator and asked the program to predict how each individual's weight loss would progress on the reduced diet. We excluded patients who admitted to straying from the diet.

The results, published in September of 2014 in the journal *Obesity,* showed that the weight loss for patients who were able to be strict with their diet was almost exactly as predicted. At an average of 13 weeks of follow up, the model predicted that average weight loss for the group would be 14 kg (+/- 9.4 kg). The observed weight loss in the 49 patients averaged 13.2 kg (+/- 8.9 kg). The correlation between predicted and actual weight loss was remarkably close ($R^2$ of .816). Basically, for everyone who could maintain this diet (and don't get me wrong, I could never maintain this diet; I've tried and lasted 6 days on my best attempt), the body worked in fairly perfect thermodynamic harmony. The results showed that a calorie did indeed seem to be a calorie.

For me, this came as a great surprise. I had made a career out of weight loss counseling and that involved being able to work with people month after month, whether things were going well or not. I didn't demand rigid adherence, but simply a good attitude and the ability to show up for the recheck appointment. I had patients who stalled on weight loss for months and months. I spent a good deal of time speculating on the biological basis of the weight loss plateau, since we do in fact, have evidence that many hormonal controls in the body respond to counteract weight loss (leptin decreases, ghrelin increases, etc). What the data in the paper told me was that, regardless of the biology, plateaus and rebound weight gain come through the patient overeating again. I had known that this was the case in theory, but to see it happening *in my clinic* was a different matter altogether.

It showed me very clearly that when we can be consistent with controlling our intake, the weight loss will not —cannot— fail. If the data in the study had come back all over the map, not in line with the computer model, I would have said, "See, the body is complex, everyone is different, we all need individual solutions relating to our unique biology." But the opposite seemed to be true: The bodies of our subjects behaved almost exactly as expected, with minimal variation. This argues that the food environment in which the individual places himself will drive health outcomes, including weight.

If we can produce such consistent weight loss with results that match a computer driven algorithm, by supplying food to our patients and monitoring them, we must ask ourselves, do we need medical degrees to treat weight problems? I continue to doubt the long term usefulness of such meal replacement programs for reasons that must now begin to sound repetitious: Weight problems occur over decades, hormonal and metabolic compensation will fight quick weight loss, and one must eventually return to a normal diet, making choices out in the world which seems geared toward overconsumption. But it does reinforce that succeeding in weight loss can occur without medical expertise. Do we need obesity experts in medicine? Certainly, but we may want to consider leaving weight loss counseling to the other professions and focus on the diagnosis and treatment of our patients' obesity-related illnesses.

**References:**

Brady, I. and Hall, KD. Dispatch from the field: Is mathematical modeling applicable to obesity treatment in the real world? *Obesity* 2014, 22(9): 1939-1941.

# Chapter 10

# The True Risk of Obesity

Many of my patients came to their first visit in the clinic and told me they were "a ticking time bomb." Men, especially, seemed to have a view of themselves as a collection of risks that, left unchecked, would, without fail, cause them to have an early heart attack. When I asked them about how dangerous obesity, specifically, was to them, many patients would tell me that it could take 10 or 20 years off their life . . . unless I could help them. Which, of course, was why they'd come to see me.

In some cases, I agreed with them. They were 30 years old, weighed 400 pounds, and had a medication list like a nursing home patient. Those guys, I worried about. But many of my weight management patients were 50-100 pounds overweight at age 50 and on just a couple of medicines. For an overweight or moderately obese person, what's the real risk? More to the point, what would be the real benefit of weight loss, in terms of additional years on the planet?

One answer comes from the work of H. Gilbert Welch and Steven Woloshin, who frequently challenge the common wisdom on medical issues. In a 2008 paper in the *Journal of the National Cancer Institute,* they assessed the absolute risk of death for U.S. adults at various ages. They showed, among other things, just how resilient we diseased, obese, Americans really are.

Taking their raw survival numbers and placing them in a simple graph form shows:

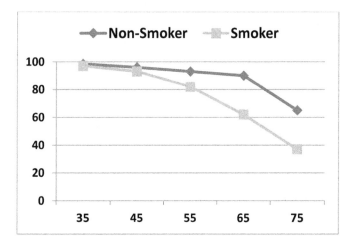

What this chart depicts is the 10 year survival, for men, at different ages. For example, if you're 35 and not a smoker, you have a 98.5% chance of making it to 45. At 45, you would re-calibrate with those that are still alive and there would be a 96% chance of living 10 more years, then 93% for the next 10, then 90% for the next. Finally, at age 75, life gets a little risky and the chance that you will live another 10 years drops to only 65%. Essentially, the 10 year risk of death is almost negligible until we get to our 70s.

Notice that the only group that needs to be separated out as having remarkably different risk is the smokers. This lifestyle choice is so dangerous that you can't talk about longevity in smokers and non-smokers together. More importantly, from my perspective, is that blood pressure, cholesterol, weight, blood sugar, all those risks we worry so much about, are nowhere to be seen. This is not because they weren't assessed for this study, they simply don't matter enough to change the statistics.

This is all comers. Everyone who lives in the U.S. Well and unwell. Light and heavy. Drinkers and non-drinkers. Everyone has, at age 55 (if they've made it to age 55) a 93% chance of living 10 more years! And if you are consciously trying to make good choices (not riding a motorcycle, not playing with handguns near your in-ground pool while intoxicated) you probably are almost *certain* to live 10 more years.

What would you expect to find if you looked harder for correlations between body mass and death statistics? I think most of us feel that being heavy is a pretty serious risk factor for death, since increased weight is associated with diabetes, heart disease, and a long list of other ailments. Most doctors would probably assume that as you move from a normal body mass index of 18.5-25, to an "overweight" BMI of 25-30 then to an "obese" BMI of greater than 30, that the risk of death would climb in a pretty linear fashion. The heavier you are, the worse off you are. *But that's simply not true.*

In a 2011 paper published in the *New England Journal,* W. Zheng and colleagues looked at health records and death statistics for over one million people over the course of 9 years. What they found is that being obese (BMI greater than 30) was associated with an increased risk of death for East Asians, but not Indians or Bangladeshis. They also found being significantly underweight (BMI less than 20) was associated with increased risk of death. But in between these two categories (weights from 130-190 pounds if you're 5' 7") the risk was flat. There was no difference in longevity for a range of body weights fluctuating 60 pounds or so.

This type of relationship, where you measure one variable against another and the extremes seem to correlate with the outcome you're interested in, is called "U-Shaped," since the lowest correlation is right in the middle. For weight, this is pretty logical: If you're very underweight, you are likely starving, frail, or ill already, so that's higher risk for death. If you're very obese, you tend to be unwell too, so no surprise there. But the "U" in the data by Dr. Zheng and colleagues was surprising, in that the bottom was essentially flat between a BMI of 20 and 30. The data seemed to suggest that having BMI 30 is no less healthy than a BMI of 20 in this population. And the Indian group and Bangledeshi group showed *no increased risk at all for the higher BMIs.* One wonders whether some of the correlation may have been lost due to the authors grouping all BMIs greater than 32.6 together. (Presumably this reflects that Asian populations have fewer people in the higher categories than are typically reported in North American populations).

This *New England Journal* study is not unique in finding that BMIs from 20-30 seem to share equal mortality risk. In a paper more about data analysis than the findings themselves, Drs. H. Gilbert Welch, Schwartz, and Woloshin looked at what they called "The exaggerated relations between diet, body weight and mortality." They demonstrated that the drawing of the "U-shaped" curve artificially minimizes differences between the BMI groups, causing the relationship to appear linear when it's not. In terms of mortality risk, the authors showed that bar graphs (and categorical

187

analysis) represented the data better than a curve and made it much more obvious that little difference exists between BMIs of 20-30.

In "BMI and Mortality: Results from a National Longitudinal Study of Canadian Adults," Heather Orpana and colleagues found, in a sample population of ~11,000 adults, that the "overweight" group was at significantly *decreased* risk of death. They also found that individuals classified as obesity Class I (BMI 30-35), were at no increased risk for mortality.

Two separate papers, both published by Katherine Flegal in *JAMA*, reinforce the idea that overweight status is *protective* for health. She found, in 2005 and in 2013, in different study populations, that the greatest longevity was attained by those with a body mass index of 27. Most recently, a large meta-analysis published by Yerrakalva et. al. in the journal *Obesity* (October 2015) showed that in 14 of 15 studies assessing the relationship between BMI and all-cause mortality, there was no association of higher BMI with death, when one accounted for age and physical activity. This *lower* risk of mortality for moderately overweight individuals has been shown so many times that we need to stop considering it a surprise and realize, again, that we aren't thinking clearly about what obesity actually *is*. Obesity is not a disease state, capable of causing early death, but a physical sign that runs with other signs and symptoms. Obesity is a product of our modern way of living, just as hypertension and high cholesterol are the products of modernity. But obesity doesn't actually cause *any* outcomes at all.

The most feared outcome we generally link to obesity is early cardiac death. In 2011, Canto and colleagues published, in *JAMA,* a study that looked at a cross-sectional view of patients who suffered a heart attack between 1994 and 2006 in U.S. hospitals. The researchers' interest was in determining how patients fared based on whether they had various risk factors, such as: hypertension, smoking, high cholesterol, diabetes or family history of heart disease. The surprising conclusion was that the fewer the number of risk factors a patient had at the time of the first heart attack, the worse they did. The researchers found that if you have a first heart attack and you are a non-smoker, non-diabetic with normal blood pressure, good cholesterol and no family history, you are *more likely to die* than someone who has all of those things.

But that's not the interesting part. The interesting part is the raw numbers that they examined. What the straight numbers show is that the group of patients you might find on any given day in the cardiac ward of a hospital looks pretty much like the general population:

52 % have high blood pressure

28 % have high cholesterol

22 % have diabetes

31 % smoke

28 % have a family history for heart disease

This is for a group of people with an average age of 66. Those numbers, aside from the smoking, (which would have been even higher if they had included former smokers) basically reflect the going rates of those factors in adults of that age group. The same is true for the breakdown on obesity:

28 % were normal weight (BMI 18-25)

36 % were overweight (BMI 25-30)

32 % were obese (BMI >30)

This demonstrates that the group recovering in the cardiac ward of a typical hospital is essentially the same as what you'd find by walking down most U.S. streets taking a random sample of adults. *So what does this mean for how we think about risk?*

We tend to over-estimate how dangerous an individual risk factor is. We don't have good statistical brains, so we try to make meaning out of things using logic rather than numbers. "Cholesterol gives you a heart attack," makes more sense to our logic-craving brains, than "high cholesterol significantly increases risk for a heart attack in some people." We certainly aren't good at keeping track of whether relationships hold going both forward and backward. For instance, thinking that high cholesterol causes heart attacks lends itself to the conclusion that all or most heart attack patients *must* have high cholesterol. But in this sample, 72% of the patients with a first heart attack had *normal* cholesterol. Let's invert the rest of the factors, as well:

48 % *did not* have hypertension

78 % *did not* have diabetes

69 % were *non*-smokers

72 % had *no family history* for heart disease

64 % were *not* obese

How would those numbers look on a public health poster or a billboard?

*"78% of all heart attack victims have normal blood sugar. Be tested today to ensure you don't have normal blood sugar."*

It's hard to scare people into doing what you want, like being screened, or joining your lifestyle program, if you can't find the risk factor to blame Why these numbers seem surprising relates to the difficulty of separating out, in our day to day thinking, the difference between *absolute* risk and *relative* risk. One example I like to use with patients that Celebrex cuts your chance of having a bleeding ulcer in half compared to ibuprofen (relative risk). The fact that it's cutting it from 3% to 1.5% (the absolute risk) is not something that the promoters of the safer medicine spend much time on, because, who would be willing to spend 25 times more for a medicine that prevents a problem from occurring almost never to . . . a little less than almost never?

Bleeding ulcers give interesting absolute numbers because they are relatively rare. Our brains want a simple rule like, "Take a lot of ibuprofen, you'll get a bleeding ulcer." But in fact, you're statistically unlikely to get a bleeding ulcer, even with the ibuprofen (97% chance of *not* having a bleeding ulcer). Our brain can't do much with, "Take a lot of ibuprofen and it's still much more likely than not that your stomach is fine." That just doesn't compute.

191

The heart attack numbers are surprising for the opposite reason: Heart attacks are so common that finding the one, absolute, cause is unlikely. In the *JAMA* study, 86 % of the heart attack patients had at least one factor that put them at increased risk. However, these risks are common in all people, so it would be difficult to find 60-year-olds without these. The breakdown looked like this:

0 risks: 14 %

1 risk: 34 %

2 risks: 32 %

3 risks: 15 %

4 risks: 4 %

5 risks: 0.4 %

Again, the risks run almost exactly opposite of our knee-jerk expectations, which would be to guess that a heart attack patient should have a greater number of risk factors. We aren't good at remembering that it gets statistically unlikely to have multiple probabilities occurring in the same person. Looking at combined probability, remember, involves multiplying decimals by other decimals, so numbers shrink quickly. The only reason the above numbers are as high as they are, is because these risks are not independent factors, but very interdependent: They run together.

This study wasn't about what causes heart attacks. There have been many of those studies and they show exactly what you'd expect: There is a linear rise in risk for heart attack as one becomes heavier, has higher blood pressure, smokes longer, etc . . . this study isn't questioning that and neither am I. However, it does show that much of the risk of a heart attack (the most dreaded outcome of all these metabolic risks we try to control by weight loss) is not subject to our control. The doctors and purveyors of tests (I'm talking about myself here) who claim they can predict and reduce risk for dreaded outcomes are focused on individual factors that simply aren't that important for most individuals. Close to half of the cases in the heart attack registry would seem like random tragedies, not controllable or preventable through diet, exercise or reducing risk factors with medication. What's strange is how well these sick people would have looked the day before their heart attack.

Why I find this interesting, in the context of our ongoing discussion of obesity and how much it matters for health, is that we can't control a lot of the risk that's out there. We want to lose weight to avoid a heart attack, but the effect weight loss has on decreasing risk of heart attack has never actually been studied. We have an assumption that most people who have a heart attack have a weight problem, but that simply isn't true; the heart attack victims have the same rate of obesity as the general population. Chance and other factors outside of our control likely have more power over our future disease risk, even in the category of lifestyle diseases, than we do ourselves.

We want there to be answers; that is our make-up. That is the story of human progress: Modern man faces mysteries and problems, scientists uncover the laws that govern the mystery, man's technology uses this knowledge to provide a solution. This does happen in medicine, but it has yet to happen in any field dealing with diet.

An oft repeated concept, when you are in medical school is that "one half of what you learn here will later be proved to be false . . . we just don't know which half yet." It's a catchy idea, but most likely untrue. The vast majority of the time in medical school is spent in the lecture hall, learning basic science that doesn't change. Where we are taught false ideas is most certainly out on the wards, when the experienced physicians show us treatment algorithms for diagnosing and treating serious ailments. At a stretch, it is possible to conceive of 20-30% of those strategies being discarded for improved methods every few decades. But the idea that half of what is taught is inaccurate seems silly and un-testable to me. Nevertheless, on the treatment side, how much of what we do is actually effective? How helpful is modern medicine?

It's a deeply held belief that physicians and the medical industry do people a world of good. We want to believe that as we grow older, regular visits to the doctor will keep us healthy. She will screen us for cancers, check our cholesterol, measure our blood pressure, adjust our medications and this will keep us alive a decade longer than we otherwise would have lived, say, a century ago. This is part of the modern ethos. We want to believe that primary care doctors prevent heart attacks and cancers by treating the risks and catching diseases before they can harm us. For some diseases, like preventing strokes by lowering blood pressure, this may be true. But for many others, such as obesity, we do not have data that show that medical treatment helps, or that it helps to the extent that the patient and doctor believe.

This is an important consideration for deciding the best treatment approach for weight problems, because the underlying assumption is that if we can describe obesity as a medical illness and unravel the biological pathology, that this will lead to medicines to "cure" it. I think that this is wishful thinking for a number of reasons, the most important of which is the complexity of regulation that I have been writing about in this book. But if we could "cure" obesity using as-yet-only-dreamed-of medications that help us lose weight, what would the real gain be? As we've just discussed, heart attack victims weigh the same as the general population and the papers on mortality show that obesity is not associated with early death, except at the very extreme.

Whether we use the term "condition" or "disease" to describe obesity, we need to reconsider what it is that we are trying to treat, prevent, measure and cure. Certainly BMI holds limited information for making policy or directing research, if the studies above are taken into consideration. Perhaps we need to insist on "adiposity" as the measurement of accumulated energy in a body. Perhaps we need only to consider metabolic manifestations, or measures of inflammation. As we've noted in several different ways in the book, it's not the fat cells themselves that are the problem; it is imbalances in our nutrition.

Nutrition does not exist solely within the human body, but as a dynamic relationship between the body and the environment. If we can redirect our attention from the individual to the environment, or at least try to focus on both simultaneously, and how they interact, I believe we can begin to find the answers to our nutritional problems.

## References:

Woloshin, S, Schwartz, LM, Welch HG. The risk of death by age, sex and smoking status in the United States: putting health risks in context. *Journal of the National Cancer Institute* 2008, 100(16): 1133.

Zheng, W, et. al. Association between body-mass index and risk of death in more than 1 million Asians. *NEJM* 2011, 364: 719-729.

Welch, HG, et. al. The exaggerated relations between diet, body weight and mortality: the case for a categorical approach. *Canadian Medical Association Journal* 2005, 172(7): 891-895.

Orpana, HM, et. al. BMI and mortality: results from a national longitudinal study of Canadian adults. *Obesity* 2012, 18(1): 214-218.

Flegal, KM, et. al. Association of all-cause mortality with overweight and obesity using standard body mass index categories. *JAMA* 2013, 309(1): 71-82.

Flegal, KM, et. al. Excess deaths associated with underweight, overweight, and obesity. *JAMA* 2005, 293(15): 1861-1867.

Yerrakalva, D, et. al. The associations of "fatness," "fitness," and physical activity with all-cause mortality in older adults: A systematic review. *Obesity* 2015, 23(10): 1944-56.

Canto, JG, et. al. Number of coronary heart disease risk factors and mortality in patients with first myocardial infarction. *JAMA* 2011, 306(19): 2120-7.

# Afterword

There is a basic formula used by "experts" who write diet books. It goes like this:

1) All diets fail.

2) Because what you've been taught about obesity is wrong.

3) I have studied the science and discovered the real truth.

4) Because I am smarter than those other guys.

5) I will share this science with you in my new book.

6) Buy My Book!

7) And you will be able to lose weight effortlessly.

My book is no exception. It follows this formula, all the way up to number 6 . . . and then just stops. It's not a joke, or a cliffhanger, dangling the final answer out there, in order to get you to buy my program that I sell elsewhere. It is the actual truth that I've found in the scientific literature. The answer to most individual's weight problem is that *there is no answer*. This could be taken as a disheartening conclusion, but I mean it to be affirming: We aren't at fault for our difficulties with weight, or if we fail when we try to diet for long periods. We can and should free ourselves from self-blame and the pressure we feel to have a different body than the one we've got.

Each chapter in this book has been based on an insight I discovered in the medical literature that helped me to understand why people are heavier now than in the past, or why weight loss is so difficult. None of these insights came from my own research. I am a clinician, so must rely on the steady flow of science as published in journals. Among the thousands of papers for which I've hit "save" or "print" over the last decade, the very few included in this book were the ones that surprised me most. When I first bumped into the literature on obesity math, for instance, I was up all night. "This is completely new!" was all I could think. "I'm an obesity doctor and *I* didn't know it worked like this, so that means . . . nobody else has heard of it either!"

This book is my attempt to "get the word out" on these few insights. They are, of course, peculiar to my way of thinking and are certainly not the only insights one could have reached after reading what I've read and observing what I've observed. For this reason, those insights are actually better framed as the "arguments" I'm making in the book. I also chose to narrow the group of arguments to ones that I believe are inter-related in such a way as to proceed in a logical sequence. But in order to make the reading somewhat manageable, transitions and a bit of narrative were added along the way, such that those key insights may have, over the course of the book, become less obvious than originally intended. For wrapping up this discussion, without wishing to insult the reader, I list them here:

—We can't fault ourselves for our weight; it's controlled by biology, not will. Ample evidence from weight loss studies shows that significant weight loss is not possible for most people.

—The extent of imbalance needed to gain 100 pounds over one's adult life is approximately 10-20 calories per day. This cannot be measured or controlled consciously.

—The path of weight gain, or loss, occurs over years and decades. Diets address days and weeks, with resumption of normal eating patterns inevitable. Very few people have actually been on a diet of a duration that would be of any use at all for long term health.

—"Low-Carb" diets have absorbed enough public attention. "Low-Carb" is an improvement over "Low-Fat," but the science of the carbohydrate hypothesis of obesity fails to address much of what controls our weight.

—The protein leverage framework shows obesity to be an ecological problem and solves many of the difficulties inherent in the calorie vs. macronutrient debate.

—Diabetes and obesity emerge in a setting of sub-optimal nutrient availability. They are not caused by gluttony, but the body's daily need for nutrition. Our food, not our conscious behavior is driving these two "diseases." If the food changes, neither condition needs to exist.

—Obesity is not an important driver of health outcomes. It doesn't drive anything at all. To the extent that the adipose tissue signals anything to the body (through its hormone production) it acts only in a manner *positive* for our health. The percentage of fat tissue in a body, or the ratio of height to weight, is simply a sort of vital sign, like blood pressure or temperature. It can indicate imbalance, but it doesn't signify disease. Taken by itself, it is almost inconsequential for long term health outcomes such as heart attack or mortality.

—Exercise helps people get fit. Getting fit and losing weight are almost entirely unrelated.

—The various weight loss industries, including medical weight loss practices such as my own, must remain ignorant, be able to live in denial of, or disagree with, some or all of these insights to continue doing what they are doing.

—Improvements in obesity rates will occur at the ecological level, through changes in the food supply which can re-align our macronutrients into better accordance with our needs. The changes needed are subtle and perhaps have already begun.

This autumn, as I've been editing these essays in an attempt to put them into some sort of logical shape and coherence, I have been taking fairly frequent walks to mull over sticky points I haven't presented well. I have been feeling very in-tune with the subtle weather changes we are having this year, one of the warmest Octobers I can recall. The leaves have been turning color so slowly and seeming to thrive on their branches, such that I began to wonder whether they would ever fall at all. They were substantially still intact at Halloween and, as it continued warm, I wondered whether this might go on. Could we have this beautiful color scheme in the forest right through till Thanksgiving perhaps? Then a couple of days ago —Wham! A hard frost came overnight, a cold, grey, terrible November day erupted with wind that shook the house windows and every single tree in the neighborhood lost its leaves in about 15 minutes. The landscape is barren and brown suddenly, as it should be this time of year. There will be a winter again this year in Iowa, no doubt about it.

In 2009, Katerina Borer and colleagues at the University of Michigan published a study on appetite. They were interested in the detailed aspects of hormonal control that act to tell the brain when it is time to eat and when to stop. Apart from the nuances discussed in the paper, I was struck by what was really the most notable finding, which was: *Eating a meal reduces hunger by 90%.* Lost in the details of how the participants perceived satiety and hunger between feedings and whether those things could be modified by exercise, or changing the type of food ingested, was the simple and overwhelming fact of nature that *we must eat regularly to feel okay.* Food is, and always will be, the most powerful appetite suppressant that we have at our disposal. No amount of tinkering in the lab to find new pathways for drug development will ever be able to change this fact. Humans are all more or less the same with regard to the fact that every five hours or so, we must eat, or endure discomfort. The fact that so many of us (doctors and patients alike) continue to address weight problems without accepting this reality leads to much unnecessary suffering by the patients who try one approach after another, failing each and blaming themselves for eating. But the drive to eat is simply a fact of normal human physiology. Winter comes to the Midwest each year; avoiding food leads to hunger. Nature is Nature, and there is no getting around it.

This needs to be the starting point for any discussion of weight. We get hungry, we eat, hunger goes away. Over the course of a lifetime, the system seems to work remarkably well. Some of us have been slightly dysregulated for a long period of time and would like to clear off the accumulated imbalance that has accrued over decades. I can't imagine an approach that could wrangle that lifelong energy regulation into quick submission without causing serious, unwanted consequences. Since weight gain comes on in increments of 10-20 calories per day over years and decades, the idea that we could undo this by reducing 1000 or 2000 calories daily strikes me as foolish. On the other hand, a moderate approach to calorie reduction, causing gradual decrease in weight, is just as unlikely to occur. As I mentioned in the first chapter, slow weight loss without intent never happens outside of serious illness. The possibility that protein leverage could exert some sort of magically beneficent effect on our bodies such that we might start to see people slim down "naturally" just by "eating better" is extremely remote. In fact, there is nothing in observable medical science that would suggest that this could occur. If there is a way for protein leverage to help individuals lose weight, it will have to be in the context of deliberate effort —as in, a "diet." On the population level, protein leverage may exert a preventative effect through changes in what's available in the shops and restaurants that we frequent. I have suggested that the nature of capitalism is to take a good idea and run with it, regardless of where the idea comes from. Given this, we may see improvement in obesity rates affecting the U.S. first, as the food innovations will likely take off here more quickly. But where we do attempt to make large scale changes to the food supply deliberately, such as through the political process, or the public policy arena, how can we carefully encourage increasing protein without causing harm?

To answer this, obesity research must broaden its scope to include an exploration of the questions, problems and possibilities suggested by the protein leverage hypothesis and the application of nutritional ecology. This field has generally been outside of the awareness of most obesity researchers. Nutritional ecology is described by David Raubenheimer as:

*". . . a branch of the biological sciences that aims to understand the role nutrition plays in mediating the relationship between animals and their environments, across timescales from short-term homeostatic responses to long-term evolutionary adaptation."*
*—Raubenheimer 2015*

Turning this branch of science toward the difficulty we humans are having with our weight will require a large, multidisciplinary effort. Luckily, the infrastructure for such an effort is already in place. Human biologists, biochemists, PhD and physician researchers of all sorts who study metabolism, have shown a fascination with the problem of obesity. The research papers pour into the journals in a flood. The workforce is already active worldwide, as the problem of obesity affects the entire globe. These scientists are primed for new insights which evoke new paths of inquiry. They need only to become aware of this burgeoning field and to begin testing the questions implied by the protein leverage hypothesis:

—What is the regulated signal from protein which causes early satiety?

—Are particular amino acids essential to this effect?

—Does the life-shortening effect of protein seen in other species apply to humans, and can this be avoided?

—Does the math of protein leverage pertain to individuals seeking weight loss?

—Do mathematical predictions reflect time periods long enough to matter for human health?

—Can the graphical models employed by Simpson and Raubenheimer be used for weight counseling, such that we can reliably predict an individual's needs?

—Which hormones or regulatory pathways mediate the protein leverage effect?

—Is there danger in purposely altering these pathways?

—Are all individuals and all human populations equally governed by protein leverage?

—Can we define optimum protein intake targets for large groups?

—How does the protein target change over the life cycle?

—Will disparities in wealth create a "protein gap" which aggravates the disadvantages in health outcomes already experienced by poorer individuals?

—And many others which relate to the unanswered questions discussed in this book. While Simpson and Raubenheimer present the protein leverage hypothesis as a ready-made conclusion from the best of their previous research, this hypothesis needs confirmation, re-confirmation, testing, probing, elaboration and articulation by many more scientists. The real value of their work, where it pertains to humans, is not to provide the solution for obesity, but to reframe the question as an ecological one and to make available a new set of tools which can serve as a foundation for a new era in obesity research. Protein does not act alone; fat and carbohydrate effects on humans can be explored more thoroughly using nutritional ecology methods as well. Other components of our nutrition, such as salt, trace minerals, and fiber, need to be examined in the same manner. The great insight that holds the potential to launch this new era of inquiry would be for human physiologists and researchers of all sorts to recognize our continuity with other species when it comes to nutritional questions. From that realization may come a new objectivity and a fresh curiosity which enables us to begin to finally unravel the mystery of human obesity.

**References:**

Borer, KT, et. al. Appetite responds to changes in meal content, whereas ghrelin, leptin and insulin track changes in energy availability. *Journal of Clinical Endocrinology and Metabolism* 2009, 94(7): 2290-98.

Raubenheimer, D. et al. Nutritional ecology of obesity: from humans to companion animals. *British Journal of Nutrition* 2015, 113: S26-39.

# Acknowledgments

I have had a tremendous amount of help learning what's presented here and, more recently, help preparing the manuscript. My patients have shared so much of their experiences, perspectives and insights while entertaining my questions, speculations and experimentation. This book comes from the journey that we took together. Alex Bassuk has been a constant support for me intellectually and has been willing to read what I write since we were kids. Natasha Gatian and Sarah Kinnison found countless errors in the manuscript. If the book is at all readable, it is thanks to them. Very busy people who have taken time to share knowledge with me include: Dan Bessesen, Kevin Hall, Stephen Simpson, David Raubenheimer, Jim Hill and Gary Taubes. The dedicated staff of the Watts Medical Library at Mercy Hospital in Cedar Rapids supplied me with difficult to obtain papers and recommended better search strategies. The MercyCare organization and its provider group understood and supported what I was doing in clinic. Aaron-Marie Thoms told me "follow your bliss" or some such cliché ten years ago, and it has worked. "VirtualDoc 3000" read and encouraged my blogging in the early days when I had fewer than 10 readers. Hank Campbell and the community at Science 2.0 have featured my writing and given me the opportunity to reach a larger, brighter, engaged online audience. My wife Tundi has put up with my obsessions remarkably well and always encouraged my flights of fancy. This is one of the few that produced something tangible. My children have given me room to read and write . . . well, they haven't given me a proper room, but part of a desk, occasional access to the laptop and much time and patience: Dexter, Esti, Phinny, Emmy —thank you.

Author photo: Estella Brady

Cover Image: iStockphoto. Leonid Andronov, image #22808382. This is a computer rendering of the hormone leptin.

Cover Design: Phineas Brady